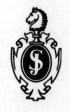

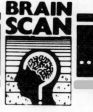

MCQ..MCQ..MCQ.. — BRAIN SCAN

David Daniels • Richard J. Hillman
Simon E. Barton • David Goldmeier

Sexually Transmitted Diseases and AIDS

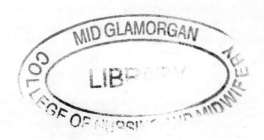

Springer-Verlag
London Berlin Heidelberg New York
Paris Tokyo Hong Kong
Barcelona Budapest

David Daniels, MA, MRCP
Senior Registrar, Department of HIV and Genito-Urinary Medicine,
St Stephen's Clinic and Westminster Hospital, London

Richard J. Hillman, BSc, MRCP, Dip. GUMed
Consultant in Genito-Urinary Medicine, The Royal London Hospital,
London

Simon E. Barton, BSc, MD, MRCOG
Consultant Physician, Department of HIV and Genito-Urinary
Medicine, St Stephen's Clinic and Charing Cross Hospital, London

David Goldmeier, MD, MRCP
Consultant Physician, Department of Genito-Urinary Medicine,
St Mary's Hospital, London

Publisher's note: The "Brainscan" logo is reproduced by courtesy of
The Editor, *Geriatric Medicine*, Modern Medicine GB Ltd.

ISBN 3-540-19762-1 Springer-Verlag Berlin Heidelberg New York
ISBN 0-387-19762-1 Springer-Verlag New York Berlin Heidelberg

British Library Cataloguing in Publication Data
Daniels, David
  Sexually Transmitted Diseases and AIDS. –
  (Brainscan MCQs Series)
  I. Title II. Series
  616.95
ISBN 3-540-19762-1

Library of Congress Cataloging-in-Publication Data
Sexually transmitted diseases and AIDS/David Daniels ... [et al.].
    p. cm. – (Brainscan MCQs)
Includes bibliographical references.
ISBN 3-540-19762-1. – ISBN 0-387-19762-1
1. Sexually transmitted diseases–Examinations, questions, etc.
I. Daniels, David, 1962– . II. Series.
    [DNLM: 1. Acquired Immunodeficiency Syndrome–examination questions.
2. Sexually Transmitted Diseases–examination questions.   WC 18 S518]
RC200.1.S478 1992
616.95'1'0076–dc20
DNLM/DLC   92-2331
for Library of Congress   CIP

Typeset by Fox Design, Bramley, Surrey
Printed by Antony Rowe Ltd., Chippenham, Wiltshire
28/3830-543210 Printed on acid-free paper

Dedication

To V and JJ
To P and GE
To HNS and ASR

Preface

The main aim of this book is to help people learn in an easy, effective and enjoyable way. It is intended to make people think, to test themselves and check the standard of their knowledge in order to pass exams as well as to improve their clinical practice for their patients.

We hope that this book will be of use to all those training in sexually transmitted diseases, doctors and nurses alike. The questions have been passed round and tried out on groups of all of these individuals, who share a common interest, yet require knowledge to different standards in order to satisfy their own curiosity and their own examiners. The recommended reading at the back of the book is suggested for those who wish to further their knowledge, check facts and pursue knowledge in the subject of sexually transmitted diseases and AIDS.

We are grateful for all our colleagues and friends who supported and helped us in ideas for questions in this edition. However, errors, differences of opinion, etc. are all our own and we trust (indeed we know) that you, the reader, will let us know of your individual feelings about the questions and answers in this book. Finally, we would like to say a special thanks to Jane Hollihead who typed the manuscript and corrected our grammar as well as to Michael Jackson who, as a very supportive publisher, cajoled us into finishing this project on time.

David Daniels
Richard J. Hillman
Simon E. Barton
David Goldmeier

Contents

1. *Historical Aspects of Genitourinary Medicine*

Q.1.1   **In the history of syphilitic infection**

    a. the first major pandemic in Europe occurred in 1495, affecting French soldiers besieging Naples

    b. the term 'Spanish Disease' was coined in 15th century Italy

    c. syphilis was first distinguished from gonorrhoea by John Hunter in 1767

    d. Philip Ricord inoculated over 2500 humans during his research on syphilis

    e. the major treatment for syphilis was arsenic, from the 16th to 18th centuries

Q.1.2   **Research landmarks in the history of sexually transmitted diseases include:**

    a. the discovery of the causative organism of gonorrhoea by Albert Neisser, a German dermatologist in 1879

    b. the discovery of the causative organism of granuloma inguinale by Augusto Ducrey

    c. the identification of *Treponema pallidum* as the cause of syphilis by Schaudinn and Hoffman in Germany in 1805

    d. the discovery of the gonococcus as a cause of proctitis by Bumm in 1884

    e. the link between syphilitic lesions of the brain and general paralysis of the insane which was discovered by Noguchi and Moore in 1913

Q.1.3   **Terms used to describe sexually transmitted infections include**

    a. Lues Maligna, which is Greek for 'spiteful plague' and describes secondary syphilis

    b. 'clap', which was first described in 1378

    c. venereal disease (Lues Venerea), which was a term first used in 1527

    d. herpes which means 'to creep' in Greek

    e. the 'magic bullet', which was a treatment for syphilis

For answers see over

Answers

A.1.1 a. T—Among the French army were Spanish mercenaries who, according to the Columbian theory, had become infected from New World natives before bringing the disease into Spain.

b. F—In Italy, syphilis was known as 'Morbo Gallico' or the 'French Disease'. In France it was called 'Le Mal de Naples' and in England 'The Spanish Disease'.

c. F—John Hunter was a Scottish surgeon who inoculated himself with pus from the penis of a patient with typical gonorrhoea. The patient coincidentally had undiagnosed syphilis, and Hunter subsequently developed both infections, leading to the mistaken deduction that they constituted only one disease.

d. T—Ricord was a 19th century French venereologist who was the first to demonstrate conclusively that syphilis and gonorrhoea were two separate entities.

e. F—Mercury was the most popular treatment for this infection during these centuries. Arsenic was not introduced until the use of Salvarsan by Ehrlich in 1909.

A.1.2 a. T

b. F—Ducrey discovered the cause of chancroid to be *Haemophilus ducreyii*, which is named after him.

c. F—This discovery was made in 1905.

d. T

e. T—Hideyo Noguchi was a renowned Japanese bacteriologist. He was also responsible for advances in knowledge concerning rabies, infantile paralysis and yellow fever. The latter of these was the cause of his death while working in West Africa.

A.1.3 a. F—It is Latin.

b. T—John of Arderne used this term to define a certain inward heat and excoriation of the urethra.

c. T—Jacque De Bethencourt in Rouen was the first to use this term.

d. T

e. T—In 1910 Ehrlich announced that arsphenamine (Salvarsan) was a 'magic bullet' which could cure syphilis in humans.

Q.1.4 **In the United Kingdom (UK), the 1916 Royal Commission on Venereal Diseases recommended that**

a. treatment should be free to all at any given institution and should not be restricted to persons resident in any particular area

b. local authorities should be empowered to supply Salvarsan or its substitutes free of charge

c. special arrangements such as evening clinics were unnecessary

d. there should be a prohibition of all advertisements of remedies for venereal diseases

e. a system of contact tracing should immediately be put into force

Q.1.5 **In the UK, the 1864 Contagious Diseases (Women) Acts were**

a. designed to reduce prostitution and sexually transmitted diseases in British garrison towns

b. used to permit the police to compel a woman found in a garrison town and declared to be a common prostitute, to undergo a forced medical examination

c. overcome by the women's movement in Britain led by Elizabeth Garratt Anderson

d. repealed in 1886

e. used to enforce screening for sexually transmitted diseases of all new army recruits

Q.1.6 **The National Health Service (Venereal Diseases) Regulation of 1974 is important because**

a. it reinforced the concept of confidentiality in persons treated for any sexually transmitted disease

b. it legalised the treatment of homosexuals with sexually transmitted diseases

c. it extended the scope of the venereal disease service so as to include all sexually transmitted diseases

d. it initiated the keeping of national statistics for syphilis and gonorrhoea

e. it declared herpes a notifiable disease

For answers see over

Answers

A.1.4   a. T

b. T

c. F—On the contrary, these were recommended for the treatment of out-patients at hours convenient to 'the working classes'.

d. T—This was designed to reduce the numbers of people being treated by unqualified practitioners, druggists and herbalists.

e. F—Partner notification was rejected by this Commission because 'any attempt to enforce notification in existing circumstances will inevitably drive a still greater proportion of the total patients suffering from these diseases ... to druggists, herbalists and other unqualified practitioners; treatment by whom is now responsible in large measure for their calamitous after consequences'.

A.1.5   a. T

b. T

c. F—This movement was led by Josephine Butler. Elizabeth Garratt Anderson opposed the campaign and believed in compulsory treatment.

d. T

e. F—The targets of this Act were women civilians.

A.1.6   a. T

b. F—Although there had never been any legal restriction against the treatment of male homosexuals, the decriminalisation of male homosexuality in 1967 did result in increased willingness of clinic attenders to admit to homosexual practices.

c. T

d. F—These statistics had been kept nationally since 1925. Figures for non-specific urethritis have been kept since 1951 and for a variety of other conditions since 1971.

e. F

Q.1.7 **The tracing of contacts of patients with sexually transmitted diseases**

a. is compulsory for patients with syphilis, gonorrhoea and chancroid in the United Kingdom

b. was compulsory for the contacts of American servicemen during the Second World War

c. is compulsory for contacts of HIV infection in the United States

d. can only be performed by Health Advisers

e. is unnecessary if a patient with gonorrhoea reliably used a condom when having sex with a named contact

For answers see over

Answers

A.1.7   a. F—Such a move was rejected by the 1916 Royal Commission on Venereal Diseases. A voluntary system, which exists up to the present day, was adopted and is not confined by law to any particular infections.

b. T—Although this system was a failure, it was designed to entail the coercive examination and treatment of contacts in the United Kingdom.

c. F—Although several schemes for partner notification of HIV have been evaluated, no compulsory schemes have so far been instigated.

d. F

e. F—Condoms afford only partial protection.

2. Human Immunodeficiency Virus (HIV) Infection

Q.2.1 **The HIV seroconversion illness**
- a. often occurs more than four months after infection
- b. may lead to cranial nerve palsies
- c. is commonly associated with an acute drop in CD4-bearing T lymphocytes
- d. may be clinically confused with glandular fever
- e. is likely to occur following needle-stick injuries involving HIV infected blood in 50% of cases

Q.2.2 **The following are Acquired Immune Deficiency Syndrome (AIDS)-defining illnesses in an HIV seropositive individual:**
- a. Oral candidosis
- b. Oral hairy leukoplakia
- c. High-grade non-Hodgkin's lymphoma
- d. Pulmonary tuberculosis
- e. Cryptococcal meningitis

Q.2.3 **The following skin conditions are more common in HIV seropositive patients than in their seronegative counterparts:**
- a. Seborrhoeic dermatitis
- b. Erythema marginatum
- c. Vitiligo
- d. Erythema nodosum
- e. Herpes simplex virus infection

Q.2.4 **The following are common oral manifestations in HIV-infected patients:**
- a. Candidosis
- b. Gingivitis
- c. Aphthous ulceration
- d. Strawberry tongue
- e. Lichen planus

For answers see over

Answers

A.2.1
a. F—It usually occurs within three months, the so-called 'window period'.
b. T—Facial nerve palsy has been described.
c. T—It may even be associated with AIDS-defining conditions such as oesophageal candida.
d. T—Investigations may show an atypical lymphocytosis, but serological tests for Epstein–Barr virus are usually negative.
e. F—Seroconversion following needle-stick injury is reported as occurring in approximately 0.5% of cases.

A.2.2
a. F—Oesophageal candidosis, or disseminated candidosis does constitute an AIDS diagnosis.
b. F—This typically occurs in AIDS-related complex (ARC).
c. T
d. F—Extra-pulmonary tuberculosis is, however, an AIDS-defining illness.
e. T

A.2.3
a. T—This is thought to be caused by *Pityrosporum* species and classically affects the eyebrows, moustache area and nasolabial folds.
b. F—This is typical of rheumatic fever.
c. F—This may be indicative of organ-specific autoimmune disorders.
d. F
e. T—Infections such as those with herpes simplex virus, human papilloma virus and molluscum contagiosum are all more common in patients with diminished cell-mediated immunity. The frequency and severity of herpes simplex infection may also be increased.

A.2.4
a. T—This is an ARC-defining sign.
b. T—Scrupulous dental hygiene and regular dental care is indicated in HIV seropositive individuals.
c. T—This can be difficult to treat, and infections such as herpes simplex, cytomegalovirus and syphilis should be excluded. There is some evidence that thalidomide is useful in recalcitrant cases.
d. F
e. F

Q.2.5   *Pneumocystis carinii* **pneumonia (PCP)**

a. can be confidently excluded if the chest x-ray is normal
b. is characteristically exacerbated if high-dose steroids are prescribed as an adjunct to antimicrobial medication
c. is typically associated with coarse crepitations on auscultation of the lungs
d. classically presents with a non-productive cough
e. is rare if the CD4 lymphocyte count is greater than $600/mm^3$

Q.2.6   **Cerebral toxoplasmosis**

a. can occur in the absence of antibodies to *Toxoplasma gondii* in the patient's serum
b. may present with a hemiparesis
c. is best confirmed by cerebrospinal fluid (CSF) examination
d. can rarely be diagnosed by computed tomographic (CT) scanning of the brain
e. is associated with a 90% mortality within two weeks of presentation

Q.2.7   **Cytomegalovirus (CMV) retinitis**

a. usually occurs when the CD4 lymphocyte count is greater than $150/mm^3$
b. is best confirmed by isolating CMV from the urine of infected individuals
c. never requires treatment if only the peripheral retina is involved
d. is associated with ophthalmological changes which disappear after treatment
e. is best treated by oral acyclovir

For answers see over

Answers

A.2.5
a. F—10%–15% of chest x-rays may be normal.
b. F—Methylprednisolone in conjunction with antipneumocystis agents has been shown to improve recovery time in patients with a $PO_2 < 8$ kPa.
c. F—Chest signs are often absent.
d. T—This is often associated with fever and progressive dyspnoea and a constricting feeling in the chest.
e. T—It is uncommon if the CD4 T lymphocyte count is greater than $250/mm^3$.

A.2.6
a. T—Although most patients will have antitoxoplasma IgG in their serum, the rising IgM titre seen in immunocompetent individuals is uncommon.
b. T—Due to the effects of the space-occupying lesion.
c. F—CSF examination is usually unhelpful and lumbar puncture is contraindicated in the presence of a space-occupying lesion in view of the risk of coning.
d. F—CT scanning of the brain classically reveals ring-enhancing lesions. Magnetic resonance imaging may be more sensitive and often reveals multiple lesions.
e. F—65%–90% of patients have an initial favourable response to therapy.

A.2.7
a. F—It is uncommon with a CD4 lymphocyte count of greater than $100/mm^3$.
b. F—Diagnosis is based on clinical findings.
c. F—Rapid disease progression may occur leading to the loss of sight.
d. F—Ophthalmoscopy in acute CMV retinitis reveals creamy white granular areas with perivascular exudates and haemorrhage. Therapy may halt progression, but retinal scarring persists.
e. F—Ganciclovir and phosphonofomate are the two agents currently in use. Although there is some evidence that high-dose oral acyclovir may have use as a prophylactic agent.

Q.2.8 **Kaposi's sarcoma**
   a. only affects cutaneous sites
   b. is never found in HIV seronegative individuals
   c. may be clinically confused with bacillary angiomatosis
   d. is a highly radioresistant tumour
   e. may regress spontaneously

Q.2.9 **Patients with AIDS have an increased risk of the following tumours:**
   a. Non-Hodgkin's lymphoma
   b. Malignant melanoma
   c. Cervical neoplasia
   d. Retinoblastoma
   e. Central nervous system (CNS) lymphoma

Q.2.10 **PCP prophylaxis**
   a. should be offered to HIV seropositive patients with CD4 lymphocyte counts consistently below $200/mm^3$
   b. is unnecessary after a single episode of PCP
   c. is rarely associated with skin rashes when co-trimoxazole is used
   d. by oral pentamidine is effective
   e. is 100% effective in fully compliant patients

Q.2.11 **The following are recognised manifestations of HIV infection:**
   a. Xeroderma
   b. Thrombocytopenia
   c. Lipomata
   d. Persistent tinea pedis
   e. Sarcoidosis

For answers see over

Answers

A.2.8   a. F—Visceral involvement is common.
            b. F—Cases have also been rarely reported in Jewish, Mediterranean, Eastern European, African and immuno-compromised individuals.
            c. T—Biopsy is desirable to confirm the diagnosis, as catch scratch disease is amenable to antibiotic therapy.
            d. F—Radiotherapy and chemotherapy are often used for treatment.
            e. T

A.2.9   a. T—B cell extranodal high grade lymphomas are more common. A role for Epstein–Barr virus in the genesis of these tumours has been postulated.
            b. F
            c. T—Studies have demonstrated an increase in both premalignant and malignant lesions, with a frequency which increases with advancing immunosuppression.
            d. F
            e. T

A.2.10 a. T—PCP rarely occurs in patients with CD4 T lymphocyte counts of greater than $250/mm^3$.
            b. F
            c. F—30% of patients develop rashes.
            d. F—Pentamidine is administered via a nebuliser or (rarely) intravenously. Other prophylactic agents include oral co-trimoxazole, dapsone and Fansidar.
            e. F—Breakthroughs have been reported with all prophylactic agents, particularly in patients with very low CD4 T lymphocyte counts.

A.2.11 a. T—Other common skin manifestations include folliculitis and seborrhoeic dermatitis.
            b. T—This is most commonly idiopathic.
            c. F
            d. T—Cutaneous fungal infections are common and may be difficult to treat.
            e. F

Q.2.12 **The following are associated with an increased risk of disease progression in HIV infected individuals:**

a. Oral candidosis
b. A high beta-2 microglobulin level
c. Multidermatomal herpes zoster
d. Penile warts
e. A leucocyte count of less than $1 \times 10^9/l$

Q.2.13 **HIV has been isolated from**

a. saliva
b. CSF
c. cervical mucus
d. whole blood
e. plasma

Q.2.14 **HIV has been described as being transmitted by**

a. vaginal intercourse
b. the sharing of needles between injecting drug users
c. kissing an infected individual
d. breast feeding
e. blood donation when disposable equipment is being used

Q.2.15 **Neurological manifestations of HIV infection include**

a. cryptococcal meningitis
b. dementia
c. an increased incidence of meningiomas
d. cranial nerve palsies
e. an increased incidence of motor neurone disease

For answers see over

Answers

A.2.12 a. T
b. T—Other laboratory parameters conferring a poor prognosis
are high serum neopterin levels, a low CD4 T lymphocyte
count, neutropenia and anaemia.
c. T
d. F
e. T

A.2.13 a. T
b. T
c. T
d. T
e. T

A.2.14 a. T
b. T
c. F—However, as HIV is demonstrable in saliva there is a
theoretical risk particularly in the presence of oral
ulceration, bleeding gums, etc.
d. T
e. F

A.2.15 a. T—Aseptic meningitis and encephalitis are also more
common in HIV seropositive individuals.
b. T—This is characterised by a triad of behavioural, motor and
cognitive dysfunction. The degree of dementia is graded
from stages 0–4; 0 being normal and 4 being a near
vegetative state.
c. F
d. T—Mononeuritis multiplex, peripheral neuropathy, neuralgic
amyotrophy and Guillain–Barré syndrome are also
described.
e. F

Q.2.16 Cryptosporidiosis in an HIV-positive patient

a. typically results in profuse watery diarrhoea
b. is best treated with ciprofloxacin
c. leads to an intense inflammatory infiltrate of the duodenal villi
d. results in deep punched out colonic ulcers
e. is associated with sclerosing cholangitis

Q.2.17 The following are common gut pathogens in patients with AIDS:

a. *Entamoeba coli*
b. *Cryptococcus neoformans*
c. *Giardia lamblia*
d. Microsporidia species
e. *Salmonella enteritidis*

Q.2.18 A child born to an HIV-infected mother

a. will inevitably be infected with HIV
b. may carry maternal HIV antibodies for longer than one year
c. may be HIV antibody negative, yet still be infected with HIV
d. is much less likely to become HIV-infected if delivered by Caesarean section
e. can be safely breast fed

Q.2.19 An HIV-infected child

a. is likely to develop symptomatic disease before its 5th birthday
b. is unlikely to develop PCP
c. is only likely to develop dementia with advanced disease
d. should be kept away from school to prevent transmission to other children
e. may benefit from zidovudine therapy

For answers see over

Answers

A.2.16 a. T—Although a minority of patients may have persistent asymptomatic infection.

b. F—There is currently no definitive treatment for cryptosporidial diarrhoea. Agents which have been tried include azithromycin, erythromycin, spiromycin and high-dose zidovudine. Paromamycin, an aminoglycoside, has shown promising early results.

c. F

d. F—This is more likely to be due to cytomegalovirus infection.

e. T—Approximately two-thirds of patients with sclerosing cholangitis will have evidence of cryptosporidiosis. However, it is currently unclear whether this association is causal.

A.2.17 a. F

b. F

c. T

d. T

e. T

A.2.18 a. F—Estimates of vertical transmission rates vary from 10% to 30%.

b. T

c. T—The diagnosis of HIV infection in children may be difficult in view of their impaired ability to mount antibody responses. Definitive proof of infection can only be obtained by direct determination of viral presence.

d. F—Method of delivery is not a major risk factor for the transmission of HIV.

e. F—Although not a common mode, HIV can be transmitted in breast milk.

A.2.19 a. T

b. F—PCP is the most common opportunistic infection in children.

c. F—Neurological and developmental abnormalities are extremely common in HIV-infected children, and may occur considerably earlier than opportunistic infections.

d. F—There is no significant risk to other children, provided that care is taken with cuts.

e. T—However, the benefits are less clear-cut than for adults.

Q.2.20 **In the diagnosis of HIV 1 infection**

    a. a negative antibody test excludes infection

    b. the Western blot method is commonly used as a screening technique

    c. p24 antigen is commonly present in the serum before specific antibody is detectable

    d. in the UK, an individual can be compelled by law to undergo testing if he is felt to have put others at risk

    e. enzyme immunoassay systems occasionally give false positive results

Q.2.21 **The following are appropriate therapies for the matched conditions:**

    a. Fluconazole–Toxoplasmosis

    b. Amphotericin B–Cryptococcal meningitis

    c. Ganciclovir–CMV retinitis

    d. Azithromycin–Oral hairy leukoplakia (OHL)

    e. Ciprofloxacin–Salmonella gastroenteritis

Q.2.22 **The following clinical situations merit recommendation of zidovudine (AZT) therapy:**

    a. Oral candidosis

    b. Kaposi's sarcoma

    c. Gingivitis

    d. A T4 count of $> 600/mm^3$

    e. Persistent tinea pedis

Q.2.23 **In a patient with PCP with a PO_2 of 6.5 kPa the following management would be appropriate:**

    a. Supplemental oxygen

    b. High-dose intravenous steroids in conjunction with anti-PCP therapy

    c. Intravenous pentamidine

    d. Ampicillin

    e. Medroxyprogesterone

For answers see over

Answers

A.2.20 a. F—With commercially available kits, HIV 1 antibodies do not become reliably detectable until 4–12 weeks after exposure. A few individuals take many months to seroconvert.

b. F—Immunoassay systems are more commonly used as they are sensitive, specific and more easily lend themselves to automation.

c. T

d. F

e. T—False-positive results can occur for technical reasons and in response to other circulating antibodies, e.g. in those with autoimmune disorders, multiparous women and people who have received multiple blood transfusions. Confirmatory testing using a second, independent method should always be performed on apparently positive results.

A.2.21 a. F

b. T

c. T

d. F—If treatment is requested, acyclovir may be helpful in the treatment of OHL.

e. T

A.2.22 a. T

b. T

c. F

d. F

e. F

A.2.23 a. T

b. T

c. T

d. F—Unless there was a suspicion of coincidental bacterial infection.

e. F

Q.2.24   Adverse effects of pentamidine include

   a. neutropenia
   b. pancreatic damage
   c. liver damage
   d. bronchoconstriction
   e. optic nerve damage

Q.2.25   When co-trimoxazole is used for the treatment of PCP

   a. side effects are uncommon
   b. 960 mg twice daily is the recommended dosage
   c. pyridoxine is usually added to the regimen
   d. Stevens–Johnson syndrome may be fatal
   e. cutaneous eruptions occur in 5% of patients

Q.2.26   In the treatment of cryptococcal meningitis

   a. dapsone/pyrimethamine is highly effective
   b. intravenous ketoconazole may be used effectively
   c. amphotericin B is frequently used
   d. post-treatment prophylaxis is used only if the patient relapses
   e. 5-flucytosine may be a useful adjunct to treatment with amphotericin B

Q.2.27   The following agents are useful in the treatment of PCP:

   a. Co-trimoxazole
   b. Pentamidine
   c. Dapsone and trimethoprim
   d. Fluconazole
   e. Primaquine and clindamycin

For answers see over

Answers

A.2.24 a. T
 b. T—This may lead to hyper and hypoglycaemia.
 c. T
 d. T
 e. F

A.2.25 a. F
 b. F—A more usual dose would be 1920 mg qds.
 c. F—Folinic acid may be added.
 d. T
 e. F—Up to 60% of patients.

A.2.26 a. F
 b. F—Penetration of the blood—brain barrier is inadequate.
 c. T
 d. F—The majority of patients will relapse when maintenance
     therapy is initiated.
 e. T—Although toxicity may limit its use.

A.2.27 a. T
 b. T
 c. T
 d. F
 e. T

3. HIV Infection: Immunology, Pathology, Microbiology

Q.3.1   **The human immunodeficiency virus (HIV 1) is**

    a. a lentivirus
    b. a retrovirus
    c. a spumavirus
    d. a DNA virus
    e. structurally similar to simian immunodeficiency virus (SIV)

Q.3.2   **HIV-1**

    a. is antigenically distinct from HIV 2
    b. only exists in one biological form
    c. is usually resistant to activated glutaraldehyde
    d. contains a major structural polypeptide in its core known as p24
    e. has a lipid-containing envelope

Q.3.3   **In the genome of HIV-1**

    a. *gag* and *env* code for structural proteins
    b. *pol* codes for a protease and an integrase
    c. the *tat* gene codes for a protein which increases production of viral structural proteins
    d. *nef* down-regulates viral gene expression
    e. *env* is the most highly conserved region

Q.3.4   **During the life cycle of HIV 1**

    a. CD4 binding sites bond specifically to p24 on the host cells
    b. gp120 is important in the virus–host cell attachment process
    c. integration of proviral DNA occurs at highly specific sites within the host DNA
    d. co-infection of the host cell with herpes viruses may reactivate transcription of latent HIV
    e. infection only occurs in T helper lymphocytes

For answers see over

Answers

A.3.1   a. T—HIV 1 is a lentivirus, which is a subfamily of retroviruses. The name lentivirus is derived from the Latin word lentus, which means 'slow', in view of the long time interval between infection and the development of clinical disease.

             b. T—The term refers to the ability of viral reverse transcriptase to transfer RNA-encoded genetic information stored within the virus into a DNA-encoded form.

             c. F—Spumaviruses, such as the human foamy virus, cause a foamy appearance in infected cells.

             d. F

             e. T

A.3.2   a. T—Although some early antibody tests failed to differentiate between the two types.

             b. F—Different HIV-1 strains show wide differences in cytopathic activity and virulence.

             c. F

             d. T

             e. F

A.3.3   a. T

             b. T

             c. T

             d. T

             e. F—This region is highly variable.

A.3.4   a. F—The T cell surface antigen CD4 binds to the viral glycoprotein gp120 before fusion of the viral envelope with the host cell.

             b. T

             c. F—Integration of the proviral DNA into the host genome seems to be at entirely random sites.

             d. T

             e. F—HIV-1 infection may occur in a variety of other cells such as macrophages and glial cells.

Q.3.5   **In the immune response to HIV 1**

    a. the first antibodies are directed against p24
    b. specific IgA is detectable in the saliva
    c. IgM levels peak at 3 weeks after exposure to the virus
    d. CD_8 bearing cytotoxic lymphocytes are important
    e. all individuals will develop HIV antibodies within 3 months of infection with the virus

Q.3.6   **Following infection with HIV**

    a. the majority of circulating lymphocytes contain viral RNA
    b. CNS damage is predominantly mediated via neuronal cell destruction
    c. a characteristic cytopathic effect with syncytial formation is frequently found in cell culture
    d. antibodies to core or *gag* proteins precede the development of antibodies to the *env* components
    e. antibodies to various HIV-1 components always remain detectable at high levels

Q.3.7   **The immune deficit of individuals infected with HIV-1**

    a. is entirely explicable in terms of depletion of CD4-bearing T lymphocytes
    b. is primarily mediated via Langerhan's cells
    c. may reduce the chance of adequate seroconversion to commercially available hepatitis B vaccine
    d. means that cholera vaccination is absolutely contraindicated
    e. involves cells of the macrophage/monocyte lineage

Q.3.8   **As a consequence of infection by HIV-1:**

    a. B cell function is only minimally impaired
    b. A polyclonal gammopathy commonly occurs
    c. Serum IgG levels are generally reduced
    d. Latent infections may be reactivated
    e. Eosinophilia frequently occurs

For answers see over

Answers

A.3.5   a. T
            b. T
            c. T
            d. T
            e. F—Although the vast majority of individuals will seroconvert to HIV within 3 months, occasional cases of more prolonged periods have been reported.

A.3.6   a. F—Only about 1 in 10 000 lymphocytes contain viral RNA.
            b. F—The majority of cells in the CNS damaged by HIV-1 are the microglial cells.
            c. T
            d. T
            e. F

A.3.7   a. F—Although loss of CD4-bearing T lymphocytes is an important component and one which is used clinically as a marker of immune depletion, other mechanisms including B cell dysfunction are involved.
            b. F
            c. T
            d. F—HIV-infected individuals tend to mount a poor response to vaccines, and are at risk of disseminated infections when live vaccines are used. Thus, the killed and toxoid-based vaccines such as cholera may be given, but not live attenuated vaccines such as oral polio.
            e. T

A.3.8   a. F
            b. T—This results in a raised total protein.
            c. F
            d. T—Infections such as toxoplasmosis and cytomegalovirus are usually due to reactivation of latent disease in HIV-infected individuals.
            e. F

Q.3.9   *Pneumocystis carinii*

a. is a virus
b. only occurs in HIV-infected individuals
c. is a major cause of pulmonary disease in HIV-positive patients
d. only causes disease in the lung
e. is best diagnosed by tissue culture

Q.3.10   **Cytomegalovirus (CMV)**

a. is a herpes virus
b. is commonly secreted asymptomatically from the cervix
c. is frequently sexually transmitted
d. in an immunocompetent individual usually causes a self-limiting infection
e. infection is more common in homosexual than in heterosexual men

Q.3.11   **CMV infection**

a. is almost universal in male homosexuals with AIDS
b. may occur as a consequence of blood transfusion
c. is always the result of reactivation of latent disease in HIV-infected individuals
d. can confidently be diagnosed on finding characteristic histological changes of biopsy specimens
e. causes a greater than four-fold rise in specific antibody titres only in a primary infection

For answers see over

Answers

A.3.9   a. F

b. F—Pneumocystis carinii pneumonia (PCP) occasionally occurs in other immunocompromised groups such as renal transplant recipients.

c. T—Unless receiving prophylactic therapy, PCP occurs in the majority of HIV-infected individuals.

d. F—There have been occasional reports of extrapulmonary pneumocystis.

e. F—A variety of staining techniques, such as modified Giemsa, silver methenamine, and immunofluorescence are the most effective.

A.3.10   a. T

b. T—Approximately 10% of third trimester pregnant women in the West shed virus in cervical secretions. The percentage is higher in the Far East.

c. T—Transmission is by intimate bodily contact.

d. T—About 40% of the adult population in Europe have serological evidence of previous CMV infection. Most infections are asymptomatic, although occasionally a mononucleosis-like illness occurs.

e. T—Seroprevalence among the male homosexual community approaches 100%.

A.3.11   a. T

b. T

c. F—Reactivation is probably the commonest cause, particularly in homosexual men, but new infections do occur.

d. T

e. F—Reactivation may also cause rising antibody titres.

Q.3.12   In the investigation of CMV infection

a. culture of the virus from bronchial lavage specimens is diagnostic of invasive CMV disease
b. a negative buffy coat culture for CMV excludes active invasive disease
c. detection of early antigen in a centrifuged blood sample is the investigation of choice
d. therapy should be withheld until laboratory results are available
e. contact tracing of sexual partners is mandatory

Q.3.13   *Cryptococcus neoformans*

a. is a protozoan
b. is found in large quantities in pigeon droppings
c. may be found in the CSF of asymptomatic HIV-positive individuals
d. infection is excluded in the absence of circulating specific serum antibodies
e. frequently causes multifocal disease in HIV-positive patients

Q.3.14   Cryptosporidiosis

a. is the commonest cause of meningitis in those infected with HIV
b. is a well-established cause of disease in HIV-negative children
c. depends on co-infection with Epstein–Barr virus before pathology occurs
d. characteristically causes a severe proctitis
e. can be reliably diagnosed by serology

For answers see over

Answers

A.3.12 a. F—CMV pneumonitis can only be conclusively diagnosed when characteristic histological changes are seen.
        b. F—CMV may fail to grow for technical reasons.
        c. T—Even under optimum conditions, CMV may take up to 6 weeks to culture. Early antigen may be rapidly detected in the buffy coat of blood using immunofluorescent antibody techniques.
        d. F—As CMV-induced damage may be irreparable, if clinical suspicion is high, specific therapy should be instituted before laboratory results are available.
        e. F—Contact tracing is of no proven benefit.

A.3.13 a. F—It is a yeast.
        b. T—The role of pigeon droppings in the epidemiology of cryptococcal infections is currently unclear.
        c. T—Cryptococcal infections may be insidious in onset.
        d. F—Antibody response is an unreliable indicator of infection. Detection of antigen is more helpful.
        e. T.

A.3.14 a. F
        b. T—Cryptosporidiosis is a common cause of diarrhoea in young children.
        c. F
        d. F
        e. F—Modified acid-fast stains are used to detect the presence of oocysts in stool samples.

4. *Human Papilloma Virus*

Q.4.1 Complete human papilloma virus (HPV) particles

a. have an envelope
b. contain double-stranded DNA in a circular arrangement
c. are abundantly present in all condylomata acuminata
d. contain histones
e. are usually found in the basal epithelial cells of infected skin

Q.4.2 Condylomata acuminata

a. are only found in the anogenital area
b. are the only manifestation of wart virus infection in the anogenital area
c. are most commonly caused by HPV types 6 and 11
d. are always the result of viral transmission during sexual intercourse
e. frequently regress during pregnancy

Q.4.3 In the treatment of penile warts:

a. Intralesional interferon α is the treatment of choice
b. Patients should abstain from sexual intercourse whilst lesions are visible
c. Fibre optic urethroscopy is mandatory to exclude the presence of urethral warts
d. Laser ablation is usually performed under local anaesthetic
e. Trichloroacetic acid helps to visualise clinically inapparent infection with HPV

Q.4.4 Podophyllotoxin paint:

a. is safe to use during pregnancy
b. is most effective against sessile anogenital warts
c. may be used in the treatment of vulval warts
d. is a recognised treatment option for flat warts of the cervix
e. must be washed off with water within two hours of application

For answers see over

Answers

A.4.1   a. F
           b. T
           c. F—HPV particles are present in only small numbers in condylomata acuminata. Common warts and plantar warts contain high numbers.
           d. T
           e. F—Viral replication occurs in basal epithelial cells. Capsid proteins are only added in more superficial layers of the epithelium.

A.4.2   a. F—Condylomata acuminata have also been described in the mouth and bladder.
           b. F—Wart virus infection of the anogenital area may be asymptomatic or cause such lesions as verruca vulgaris and sessile warts.
           c. T
           d. F—There is evidence of perinatal transmission.
           e. F—Condylomata acuminata frequently increase in size and number during pregnancy.

A.4.3   a. F
           b. F—Sexual intercourse may continue during treatment, provided condoms covering the lesions are used to prevent further spread.
           c. F—The majority of urethral warts are visible at the meatus. Urethroscopy is indicated if the clinical state suggests more proximal spread.
           d. T
           e. F—3%–5% acetic acid is usually used for this purpose, although the sensitivity and specificity of this technique are low.

A.4.4   a. F
           b. F—It is most effective against condylomata acuminata.
           c. T—Women need clear instructions where to apply the treatment and usually a mirror is necessary to visualise the lesions properly.
           d. F
           e. F—Washing after application is not required unlike the recommendation after use of podophyllin paint.

Questions

Q.4.5 **In cryotherapy of anogenital warts:**

a. Liquid nitrogen freezes to a lower temperature than systems using carbon dioxide
b. Podophyllotoxin application may be used in conjunction
c. Two freeze–thaw cycles lead to a more rapid resolution of lesions than one freeze–thaw cycle
d. Local anaesthesia is not usually necessary
e. Pregnancy is not a contraindication

Q.4.6 **In the diagnosis of anogenital HPV infections:**

a. Culture using human embryonic lung cell lines is the most commonly used technique
b. The detection of specific IgG to the L_1 capsid protein is diagnostic of a recent infection with HPV
c. Biopsy of at least one visible lesion is mandatory
d. The presence of koilocytes in a Papanicolaou smear is highly suggestive of cervical involvement
e. A finding of perianal warts in a woman is indicative of previous receptive anal intercourse

Q.4.7 **Genital warts:**

a. In children are diagnostic of sexual abuse
b. Show different morphologies depending on the type of HPV present
c. Tend to be most commonly found at sites of maximum trauma during sexual intercourse
d. Only occur in uncircumcised men
e. May be treated effectively with acyclovir cream

For answers see over

Answers

A.4.5   a. T
           b. T
           c. T
           d. T
           e. T—Cryotherapy and trichloroacetic acid are safe in pregnancy.

A.4.6   a. F—Clinical diagnosis is usually adequate. Tissue culture systems are generally ineffective, as HPV requires differentiating epithelium within which to multiply.
           b. F—Serological responses are currently unreliable in the diagnosis of HPV infections.
           c. F—Biopsy is only necessary for atypical lesions.
           d. T
           e. F—Perianal warts may arise in women (and occasionally men) through passive transfer of virus particles from the genital region.

A.4.7   a. F—Perinatal transmission may occur, but sexual abuse should always be excluded.
           b. F
           c. T
           d. F
           e. F

5. *Genital Herpes*

Q.5.1   Common clinical features of primary genital herpes simplex virus (HSV) infection include

a. fever
b. meningitis
c. erythema marginatum
d. dysuria in women
e. hepatitis

Q.5.2   The differential diagnosis of genital HSV infection includes

a. Behçet's disease
b. lymphogranuloma venereum
c. Reiter's syndrome
d. Stevens–Johnson syndrome
e. late latent syphilis

Q.5.3   The diagnosis of HSV infection may be reliably confirmed by

a. light microscopy of a Gram-stained smear
b. viral culture
c. cytological examination using a Papanicolaou smear
d. electron microscopy
e. direct immunofluorescence staining of ulcer material

Q.5.4   The following systemic antiviral drugs are effective in the treatment of HSV:

a. Alpha interferon
b. Acyclovir
c. Idoxuridine
d. Vinblastine
e. Phosphonoformate

For answers see over

Answers

A.5.1   a. T
           b. T—This occurs in approximately 36% of women and 13% of men with primary genital infection.
           c. F—Although erythema multiforme may occur.
           d. T—This can contribute to urinary retention, in addition to an autonomic neuropathy.
           e. F—This is uncommon but can occur.

A.5.2   a. T
           b. T
           c. T—Circinate balanitis may resemble herpetic lesions.
           d. T
           e. F—By definition, late latent syphilis is asymptomatic.

A.5.3   a. F
           b. T
           c. F—This is an insensitive (although specific) diagnostic method.
           d. T
           e. T

A.5.4   a. F
           b. T
           c. F—Systemic toxicity (bone marrow suppression and hepatotoxicity) limits idoxuridine to topical use.
           d. F
           e. T—Phosphonoformate (Foscarnet) has been used to treat acyclovir-resistant HSV in patients with AIDS.

Q.5.5 **In patients with genital HSV infections:**

    a. An increased risk of cervical carcinoma has been described in those with antibodies to HSV-2

    b. *In vitro* resistance to acyclovir can only occur in HSV-2

    c. No effective vaccine for the prevention of transmission of HSV to uninfected contacts is yet available

    d. There is approximately a 10% mortality in neonates with CNS involvement

    e. Fifty per cent of the DNA content of HSV-2 is similar to that in HSV-1

Q.5.6 **Primary genital HSV infection**

    a. is the same as 'first-attack' genital herpes

    b. may result in cervical infection in 25% of female cases

    c. due to HSV-1 leads to more frequent recurrences than infection by HSV-2

    d. may lead to urinary retention

    e. is rarely associated with inguinal lymphadenopathy

Q.5.7 **HSV**

    a. is a DNA virus

    b. has an envelope containing five glycoproteins

    c. contains a complex RNA genome with molecular weight of 100×10^6 daltons

    d. possesses an octahedral capsid

    e. is a retrovirus

Q.5.8 **The following are herpesviruses:**

    a. Cytomegalovirus

    b. Hepatitis C

    c. Epstein–Barr virus

    d. *Mycoplasma pneumoniae*

    e. Varicella zoster

For answers see over

Answers

A.5.5   a. T—Although this association is not thought to be causal.

b. F—*In vitro* resistance to acyclovir occurs in both HSV-1 and HSV-2, although the clinical importance of this is currently unclear.

c. T

d. F—The mortality rate is approximately 50%, even with treatment.

e. T

A.5.6   a. F—'First-attack' genital herpes occurs when the patient has previously been exposed to HSV prior to acquiring their genital infection. Primary genital herpes occurs in patients with genital infection but no previous exposure to any HSV.

b. F—Over 80% of women with genital HSV have evidence of cervical involvement.

c. F—Primary genital herpes due to HSV-2 is more likely to result in recurrences.

d. T—Urinary problems are common in patients with primary or 'first-attack' genital herpes. This may be due to reflex spasm associated with painful lesions, or autonomic nerve dysfunction.

e. F—Over 80% of male and female patients will have bilateral inguinal lymphadenopathy.

A.5.7   a. T

b. T

c. F—It has a DNA genome.

d. F—It is icosahedral.

e. F

A.5.8   a. T

b. F

c. T

d. F

e. T

Q.5.9 **The management of recurrent genital herpes may usefully include**

a. regular saline washes
b. idoxuridine applications
c. counselling of the patient
d. acyclovir cream
e. ultraviolet light therapy

Q.5.10 **Genital herpes simplex infection in pregnancy**

a. is associated with spontaneous abortion
b. is associated with cleft palate of the fetus
c. is associated with preterm labour
d. necessitates fetal delivery by Caesarean section
e. can rarely result in a fatal disseminated infection in the mother

Q.5.11 **Asymptomatic shedding of HSV**

a. occurs in up to 5% of healthy adults in their oral secretions
b. has been detected in 24% of cervicovaginal secretions of female university students
c. from the cervix has never been observed to persist for longer than two weeks in a healthy woman
d. occurs in up to 7% of the genital secretions in women attending a sexually transmitted disease clinic
e. from the genitals accounts for the majority of cases of neonatal HSV infection in the UK

Q.5.12 **The following techniques are useful for typing HSV isolates:**

a. Restriction endonuclease analysis
b. Microneutralisation using rabbit antisera
c. Electron microscopy
d. Serological testing for specific IgA
e. Pock size on the chorioallantoic membrane where HSV-1 produces larger pocks

For answers see over

Answers

A.5.9   a. T
          b. F—Are expensive and clinically ineffective.
          c. T
          d. T—But success depends on starting treatment very early on
               in the attack, and clinical improvement is slight.
          e. F—Sunbathing may provoke an attack.

A.5.10 a. T
          b. F
          c. T
          d. F—If there are no lesions at term on the vulva or cervix and
               the membranes are intact, vaginal delivery may be
               allowed. Such a neonate should be closely followed for
               signs of neonatal herpes for a number of weeks.
          e. T

A.5.11 a. T
          b. F—A study of asymptomatic female university students in
               America found a detection rate of 0.5%.
          c. F—Continuously positive cervical cultures have been
               identified for up to one month.
          d. T
          e. F

A.5.12 a. T—HSV-1 and HSV-2 can be separated unambiguously using
               this technique.
          b. T
          c. T—The production of filaments by HSV-2 is used to
               distinguish it from HSV-1 by this technique.
          d. F—IgG to glycoprotein G has been shown to be type specific
               and is used for this purpose.
          e. F—HSV-2 produces pocks of > or = 1 mm where as HSV-1
               produces pocks of < or = 0.75 mm.

Q.5.13   Acyclovir

a. was discovered in 1978
b. is an acyclic purine nucleoside analogue, which inhibits the RNA polymerase of HSV
c. requires thymidine kinase to produce acyclovir monophosphate within herpes-infected cells for it to be effective
d. is not phosphorylated by thymidine kinase in normal human cells
e. is excreted by glomerular filtration and renal tubular excretion

Q.5.14   The following are correct concerning the pharmacology of acyclovir:

a. At therapeutic doses 60% of acyclovir is absorbed from the gastrointestinal tract
b. Peak serum levels are found within two hours after an oral dose
c. Acyclovir is rapidly degraded into several active metabolites
d. Acyclovir is 95% protein bound in serum
e. Acyclovir may crystallise within the kidney tubules causing renal failure

Q.5.15   The reported incidence of neonatal HSV infection:

a. in the United States is greater than that in the United Kingdom
b. is greater in higher socioeconomic groups
c. is due to HSV-2 in more than 80% of cases
d. is acquired from a person other than the mother in up to one-third of cases
e. Is much higher and more severe in premature neonates

For answers see over

Answers

A.5.13 a. T
          b. F—It is the inhibition of DNA polymerase which exerts the antiviral effect.
          c. T
          d. T—Although a small amount of phosphorylated acyclovir is produced in normal cells by an unidentified cellular enzyme system.
          e. T

A.5.14 a. F—Less than 30% of an oral dose is absorbed.
          b. T
          c. F—The majority of acyclovir is excreted unchanged through the kidneys.
          d. F—Less than 20% is protein bound.
          e. T—In patients with impaired renal function the doses of acyclovir need to be reduced.

A.5.15 a. T—By ten-fold.
          b. F—Lower socioeconomic groups have a greater incidence of infection.
          c. T
          d. T
          e. T

6. *Hepatitis A/B/C/D*

Q.6.1   Hepatitis A infection

 a. leads to chronic liver disease in approximately 1% of cases
 b. is transmitted via the orofaecal route
 c. has an incubation period of six weeks to six months
 d. leads to fulminant hepatic failure in approximately 5% of cases
 e. is best diagnosed by electron microscopic examination of stool specimens for virus particles

Q.6.2   In acute hepatitis B infection

 a. the initial immune response is IgG anticore antibody
 b. a prolonged prothrombin time is a useful prognostic indicator
 c. antimitochondrial antibodies are present in up to 40% of patients
 d. patients are no longer infectious as soon as jaundice appears
 e. approximately 5% of patients will progress to chronic infection

Q.6.3   The following are associated with hepatitis B infection:

 a. Polyarthralgia
 b. Polyarteritis nodosum
 c. Hepatic adenomata
 d. Rheumatoid arthritis
 e. Hepatocellular carcinoma

Q.6.4   Hepatitis B vaccination

 a. consistently confers lifelong immunity
 b. is most effective if given by subcutaneous injection
 c. is highly effective in HIV-seropositive individuals
 d. may lead to acute hepatitis B infection in a minority of recipients
 e. confers immunity in 90% of people after a single injection

For answers see over

Answers

A.6.1 a. F—Chronicity may follow hepatitis B and C infection but not hepatitis A.
b. T
c. F—The incubation period is six days to six weeks.
d. F—This complication occurs in less than 1% of cases.
e. F—Detection of IgM class antibodies to hepatitis A is the investigation of choice.

A.6.2 a. F—The development of IgM class antibody to core protein is the initial immune response, followed by surface antibody production.
b. T—This implies severe hepatic dysfunction.
c. F—This is typical of primary biliary sclerosis.
d. F—Infectivity may persist through and beyond the icteric phase.
e. T—Chronic carriage is defined as the persistence of hepatitis B surface antigen for at least six months following the acute infection. Men are 2–3 times more likely to develop this than women.

A.6.3 a. T—This typically occurs during the acute stage of infection.
b. T
c. F
d. F
e. T

A.6.4 a. F—After vaccination, periodic measurement of hepatitis B surface antibodies is recommended. A level of less than 10 international units/ml indicates that a booster dose of vaccine is required.
b. F—Intramuscular injection into the deltoid is the most efficacious route. Intradermal vaccination is also possible.
c. F—Induction of hepatitis B surface antibody is impaired.
d. F
e. F—Three injections are necessary to achieve this level of protection. The recommended regimen involves vaccination at time 0, 1 month and six months.

Q.6.5   Delta hepatitis

a. is an incomplete RNA virus
b. always requires co-existent hepatitis B infection in order to infect hepatocytes
c. is more common in homosexual men than in injecting drug users
d. may be spread parenterally
e. superinfection may lead to an acute exacerbation of hepatitis in patients with chronic hepatitis B infection

Q.6.6   Hepatitis B

a. infection is caused by a DNA virus of the hepadna group
b. infection may cause symptoms indistinguishable from drug-induced hepatitis
c. is usually transmitted via the enteric route
d. infection cannot occur twice in an individual
e. may be prevented by passive immunisation using hyperimmune gamma globulin

Q.6.7   The following groups are at risk of hepatitis B infection:

a. Practising male homosexuals
b. Injecting drug users
c. Orthopaedic surgeons
d. Heterosexual blood donors, where disposable sterile equipment is used
e. Female prostitutes

Q.6.8   Hepatitis C

a. infection may lead to chronic liver disease
b. has a similar mode of transmission to hepatitis A
c. is seen in less than 20% of haemophiliacs
d. leads to an acute antibody response typically within one week
e. is an RNA virus

For answers see over

Answers

A.6.5 a. T
        b. T
        c. F—It is more common in injecting drug users.
        d. T
        e. T—It also predisposes to chronic active hepatitis and cirrhosis.

A.6.6 a. T
        b. T—Viral, drug-induced and alcohol-induced hepatitis may be indistinguishable on clinical grounds.
        c. F
        d. F—Recrudescence of infection has been described in HIV-seropositive patients who were previously hepatitis B surface-antibody positive. Reinfection has also been reported.
        e. T—Hyperimmune gamma globulin is recommended immediately following exposure to hepatitis B in non-immune patients. Active vaccination against hepatitis B should be started simultaneously.

A.6.7 a. T
        b. T
        c. T
        d. F
        e. T
Hepatitis B is spread by the parental, sexual and vertical route. Vaccination is recommended for health care workers, injecting drug users, male homosexuals and those likely to have sexual intercourse in areas of high endemicity.

A.6.8 a. T—Hepatitis C accounts for 70%–90% of post-transfusion hepatitis (previously known as non-A non-B hepatitis). Like hepatitis B, it may lead to chronic infection and cirrhosis.
        b. F—The routes of transmission are similar to hepatitis B.
        c. F—60%–90% of haemophiliacs who have received commercial Factor VIII have antibodies to hepatitis C.
        d. F—Using current methods, antibodies may not be detectable to hepatitis C for several months.
        e. T

Q.6.9 **The treatment of chronic hepatitis B infection may usefully include**

a. interferon
b. zidovudine
c. acyclovir
d. azithromycin
e. medroxyprogesterone

For answers see over

Answers

A.6.9   a. T—Alpha interferon has been shown to increase the rate of seroconversion from hepatitis B 'e' antigen to hepatitis B 'e' antibody positivity.

      b. F

      c. F

      d. F

      e. F

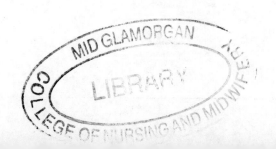

7. Syphilis

Q.7.1 *Treponema pallidum*

a. can only be distinguished from *T. pertenue* and *T. carateum* on the basis of morphological differences
b. can be readily visualised by Gram staining of material obtained from the base of a chancre
c. is an obligate parasite
d. cannot be maintained in continuous culture in vitro
e. can be found in large quantities in gummas

Q.7.2 **Primary syphilis**

a. occurs in approximately one-third to one-half of sexual contacts of an infected individual
b. is always symptomatic
c. has a mean incubation time of approximately one week
d. does not occur in those with a previous history of treated syphilis
e. is characteristically associated with the appearance of an ulcer at the site of inoculation

Q.7.3 **Chancres of primary syphilis**

a. are characteristically painful
b. typically last for at least 3 months
c. only recur as a result of reinfection
d. are rarely associated with regional lymphadenopathy
e. only resolve after appropriate antibiotic treatment

Q.7.4 **In the diagnosis of primary syphilis:**

a. serological tests are useless
b. the presence of pathogenic treponemes can be reliably established by performing a dark-ground examination of oral chancres
c. direct immunofluorescence is a more sensitive means of detecting *T. pallidum* than dark-ground examinations
d. it is safe to give co-trimoxazole while the diagnosis is being established
e. a negative fluorescent treponemal antibody (FTA) test taken from a patient with a genital ulcer excludes a diagnosis of syphilis

For answers see over

Answers

A.7.1   a. F—*T. pallidum*, *T. pertenue* and *T. carateum* are morphologically and serologically indistinguishable.

            b. F—Because of the narrow width of the treponemes, dark-field examination is necessary.

            c. T

            d. T

            e. F—Treponemes are only found in large numbers in lesions of primary and secondary syphilis.

A.7.2   a. T

            b. F

            c. F—The mean incubation time is 3 weeks with a range of 10–90 days.

            d. F—Although a degree of immunity does develop it is unlikely to be protective against subsequent attacks.

            e. T

A.7.3   a. F

            b. F—Chancres typically last for 3–6 weeks without treatment.

            c. F—Rarely there is a relapse of the primary chancre (a chancre 'redux') at the site of the primary lesion.

            d. F—Regional lymphadenopathy is common.

            e. F—Resolution always eventually occurs.

A.7.4   a. F

            b. F

            c. T

            d. T

            e. F

Questions

Q.7.5   Secondary syphilis

    a. is commonly accompanied by *T. pallidum* bacteraemia
    b. typically causes a pruritic, maculopapular rash
    c. is a cause of alopecia
    d. classically is associated with aphthous ulceration in the mouth and other mucous membranes
    e. is a recognised cause of the nephrotic syndrome

Q.7.6   In the investigation of secondary syphilis

    a. dark-ground analysis of papillomatous lesions may be helpful
    b. positive treponemal serology occurs in approximately 100% of cases
    c. a rising titre of the venereal disease research laboratory (VDRL) test is diagnostic
    d. the prozone phenomenon may lead to a false positive VDRL
    e. the VDRL test is a specific treponemal test

Q.7.7   The following treatments are acceptable in the treatment of early syphilis:

    a. Benzathine penicillin 2.4 Miu intramuscularly (i.m.) on two occasions, six days apart
    b. Doxycycline 100 mg orally twice daily for one week
    c. Ciprofloxacin 250 mg orally twice daily for one week
    d. Erythromycin 500 mg orally twice daily for 2 weeks
    e. Ceftriaxone 250 mg i.m. once daily for 10 days

Q.7.8   The Jarisch–Herxheimer reaction

    a. is associated with the production of Donath–Landsteiner antibodies
    b. is most common in individuals with tertiary syphilis
    c. may be associated with preterm labour
    d. can result in myocardial infarction
    e. is most likely to occur if penicillin is used

For answers see over

Answers

A.7.5   a. T

b. F—The rash of secondary syphilis is typically non-pruritic, although occasionally pruritis does occur.

c. T

d. F—The mucosal ulcers, or 'mucous patches' of secondary syphilis are painless. 'Aphthous' means burning.

e. T—Immune complex glomerulonephritis resulting in the nephrotic syndrome occasionally occurs.

A.7.6   a. T—Condylomata lata may be teeming with treponemes.

b. T—False negative serology may rarely occur.

c. T—A fourfold rise in titre is considered diagnostic.

d. F—This results in a false negative VDRL.

e. F—Acute and chronic biological false positives occur.

A.7.7   a. T

b. F

c. F

d. T

e. T

The CDC guidelines suggest the following treatments are adequate for the management of early syphilis (less than 1 year duration):

benzathine penicillin 2.4 Miu i.m. on one occasion

doxycycline 100 mg orally twice daily for two weeks

erythromycin 500 mg four times daily for 2 weeks

ceftriaxone 250 mg once daily for 10 days

ciprofloxacin has only slight activity against *T. pallidum*

A.7.8   a. F

b. F—It is more common in those with early syphilis, but more dangerous in those with tertiary syphilis.

c. T

d. T

e. F—It is independent of the type of therapy.

8. *Gonococcal Infection*

Q.8.1   *Neisseria gonorrhoeae*

a. can be differentiated from *N. meningitidis* by sugar fermenta-
tion tests
b. is best cultured on Sabouraud's medium
c. is an anaerobic Gram-negative coccus
d. is highly sensitive to metronidazole
e. is highly resistant to drying

Q.8.2   **Urethral gonococcal infection**

a. can be definitively diagnosed by the finding of Gram-
negative intracellular diplococci
b. may be asymptomatic in up to 10% of heterosexual men
c. cannot be acquired by oral sex
d. may result in a periurethral abscess
e. usually undergoes spontaneous remission after two weeks

Q.8.3   **Rectal gonorrhoea**

a. only occurs in homosexual males
b. causes symptoms in at least 90% of male patients
c. requires intravenous antibiotics for treatment
d. may cause diarrhoea
e. may present with tenesmus and muco-pus streaking of the
stool

Q.8.4   **Gonococcal pharyngitis**

a. commonly results in a severe purulent tonsillitis
b. is diagnosed by a Gram-stained smear from the pharynx
c. is best treated by ampicillin and probenecid as a single dose
d. can lead to disseminated gonococcal infection
e. may resolve spontaneously

For answers see over

Answers

A.8.1 a. T—*N. gonorrhoeae* ferments glucose, *N. meningitidis* ferments maltose and glucose.
    b. F—Sabouraud's is a specialised fungal growth medium. *N. gonorrhoeae* has exacting growth requirements requiring an atmosphere rich in carbon dioxide and a medium such as lysed blood agar.
    c. F—It is an aerobic Gram negative coccus.
    d. F
    e. F—It is highly sensitive to desiccation.

A.8.2 a. F—A presumptive diagnosis, confirmed by culture can be made on microscopy. *N. meningitidis* may occasionally cause genital infection.
    b. T
    c. F
    d. T—This is one of the local complications of gonorrhoea.
    e. F—But prolonged infection may become less symptomatic.

A.8.3 a. F
    b. F—Studies vary from 30% to 82% of male homosexuals.
    c. F—Single dose oral ciprofloxacin therapy is effective.
    d. T
    e. T

A.8.4 a. F—It is usually asymptomatic with minimal signs.
    b. F—Commensal *Neisseria* species may cause confusion and culture is mandatory.
    c. F—More prolonged therapy is necessary.
    d. T
    e. T—Up to 100% resolve within 12 weeks of infection.

Q.8.5   **Disseminated gonococcal infection**

   a. commonly presents with erythema nodosum
   b. is more common with beta-lactamase-producing strains of the gonococcus than with penicillin-sensitive strains
   c. may present with a small joint polyarthropathy
   d. often leads to profound thrombocytopenia and septicaemic shock
   e. is best diagnosed by Gram-staining aspirate from the affected joints

Q.8.6   **The site(s) most likely to yield *N. gonorrhoeae* in infected women are:**

   a. the cervix
   b. the urethra
   c. the rectum
   d. the pharynx
   e. posterior vaginal fornix

For answers see over

Answers

A.8.5   a. F—The typical skin lesions are necrotic pustules.
            b. F—Disseminated gonococcal infection is usually caused by penicillin-sensitive strains.
            c. T
            d. F—This is more often seen with *N. meningitidis.*
            e. F—Diagnosis is best made by sampling of genital and pharyngeal sites, however Gram stain and culture of joint aspirate and blood cultures should be performed.

A.8.6   a. T
            b. T
            c. T
            d. T
            e. F

Isolation rates of N. gonorrhoeae in female orogenital infection

Urethra 70%–90%
Rectum 35%–50%
Pharynx 10%–20%
Cervix > 90%
Swabs from the posterior vaginal fornix are unreliable, as the gonococcus preferentially infects columnar epithelium.

9. *Chlamydia*

Q.9.1   *Chlamydia trachomatis*

a. can be detected by Gram staining of swabs taken from infected sites
b. will grow on modified horse blood agar under microaerophilic conditions
c. causes characteristic lysis of McCoy cell lines
d. has been implicated in adult respiratory disease
e. may rarely be a zoonosis

Q.9.2   *C. trachomatis*

a. is a facultative intracellular parasite
b. is classified as a bacterium
c. can only be successfully propagated in cell culture
d. exists as two different, morphologically distinct forms
e. may be part of the normal vaginal flora

Q.9.3   **Chlamydial cervicitis**

a. can be reliably diagnosed from pus scores of a Gram-stained cervical swab
b. is best treated with ciprofloxacin
c. is usually asymptomatic
d. always causes pathognomonic cytological changes on a Papanicolaou smear
e. is caused by infection of the squamous epithelium

Q.9.4   *C. trachomatis*

a. can be isolated from the urethras of approximately 95% of men with non-gonococcal urethritis
b. is reliably detected by antigen-based enzyme-linked immunosorbent assay (ELISA) tests
c. is the commonest cause of non-gonococcal urethritis in homosexual men
d. is a significant cause of pneumonitis in immunocompetent adults
e. may be transmitted by orogenital contact

For answers see over

Answers

A.9.1   a. F

        b. F—It can only be grown in cell culture.

        c. F—McCoy cells are used to culture *C. trachomatis*. Identification is then usually performed by Giemsa, iodine or immunofluorescent staining.

        d. T—Although this may be due to serological cross reactivity with *C. pneumoniae*.

        e. F

A.9.2   a. F—It is an obligate parasite.

        b. T

        c. T

        d. T—Extracellular elementary bodies and metabolically active intracellular reticulate bodies.

        e. F

A.9.3   a. F

        b. F—Ciprofloxacin is effective against *C. trachomatis* but has no advantage over cheaper drugs such as the tetracyclines.

        c. T

        d. F—Inflammatory cytological changes are seen, but are neither sensitive nor specific for cervicitis caused by *C. trachomatis*.

        e. F—*C. trachomatis* colonises columnar epithelium.

A.9.4   a. F—About 40% of cases of non-gonococcal urethritis are associated with urethral colonisation by *C. trachomatis*.

        b. T—Antigen-based ELISA tests are frequently used in clinical practice. Direct immunofluorescence and cell culture techniques are also used.

        c. T

        d. F

        e. T

Q.9.5 Infection with *C. trachomatis*

a. is an extremely rare occurrence of the rectal mucosa
b. is a frequent cause of epididymitis in sexually active heterosexual men
c. is a cause of the urethral syndrome in women
d. is a recognised cause of Bartholinitis
e. is more common in women with cervical ectopy

Q.9.6 Clinically apparent urogenital infection with *C. trachomatis*

a. normally develops in men within 2 weeks after exposure
b. does not occur in pregnant women
c. may result in ocular disease through spread of infected genital secretions
d. only occurs once in immunocompetent individuals, due to the development of cell-mediated immunity
e. is always sexually transmitted

Q.9.7 In the treatment of genital infection with *C. trachomatis*

a. penicillin is highly effective
b. 4-quinolones have no significant antimicrobial activity
c. macrolides are effective
d. tetracyclines play a useful role
e. tetracycline resistance is a common cause of treatment failure

Q.9.8 In the investigation of urogenital infection with *C. trachomatis*

a. serial specific antibody titres are usually used to establish the diagnosis
b. a single negative antigen-based ELISA test reliably excludes infection
c. direct immunofluorescence methods are generally more sensitive and specific than ELISA methods
d. cell culture techniques are generally unhelpful
e. test of cure should always be performed using an ELISA method 7 days after initiating therapy

For answers see over

Answers

A.9.5   a. F—It is a significant cause of proctitis in homosexual men.
             b. T
             c. T
             d. T
             e. T—Possibly as a consequence of the increased area of columnar epithelium available for colonisation with *C. trachomatis*.

A.9.6   a. T
             b. F
             c. T
             d. F—Repeated infections at the same site are possible.
             e. T

A.9.7   a. F
             b. F—Ofloxacin is highly effective against *C. trachomatis*.
             c. T—Erythromycin is a useful drug, although requires treatment for at least a week. Azithromycin seems to be effective in a single dose.
             d. T
             e. F—Tetracycline resistance is not a clinical problem.

A.9.8   a. F
             b. F—Repeat testing is indicated if clinical suspicion is high.
             c. T—Although the local availability of skills usually governs which tests are used.
             d. F—Cell culture techniques are reasonably sensitive and highly specific, but are technically demanding.
             e. F—Antigen may still be present at this stage, in the absence of viable organisms, thus giving a false positive result. At least two weeks should elapse before a test of cure can be performed using antigen-based methods.

Q.9.9 **Reiter's syndrome**

a. only occurs after chlamydial urethritis
b. is more common in men with the HLA-B27 haplotype
c. is related to infection with specific antigenic strains of *C. trachomatis*
d. is rarely associated with a progressive, destructive arthropathy
e. may be associated with retinal lesions

Q.9.10 **When taking genital samples for the detection of *C. trachomatis***

a. it is important to remove mucus and debris from the cervix before sampling
b. an Aylesbury spatula is particularly useful for obtaining cervical material
c. it is important to refrigerate samples while awaiting analysis by antigen detection methods
d. menstruation renders antigen detection methods unreliable
e. male urethral samples should be taken from at least 4 cm proximal to the meatus

Q.9.11 **In heterosexual men attending STD clinics**

a. a urethral smear is unnecessary unless symptoms of urethritis are present
b. non-gonococcal urethritis (NGU) can be confidently diagnosed in the absence of evidence of gonorrhoea and in the presence of > 5 pus cells per high power field from a urethral swab and threads in the first sample of the two glass urine test
c. NGU can be excluded in any man if there are < 5 pus cells per high power field from a urethral swab
d. > 5 pus cells per high power field from a urethral swab is always diagnostic of NGU
e. time since last past urine is an important variable in urethral microscopic findings

For answers see over

Answers

A.9.9   a. F—It may also follow gut infection with Shigella spp., *Salmonella* spp., *Campylobacter* spp. and *Yersinia enterocolitica*
            b. T
            c. F
            d. T
            e. F

A.9.10   a. T
            b. F—When sampling for *C. trachomatis*, wooden spatulae should be avoided as they may be toxic to the organism.
            c. F
            d. F
            e. T

A.9.11   a. F
            b. T
            c. F—Repeat testing may be necessary if clinical suspicion is high. The patient may be incubating infection or have recently passed urine.
            d. F—This may occur in cases of balanitis and urinary tract infection.
            e. T

Q.9.12 *Mycoplasma hominis*

    a. is the same organism as *Ureaplasma urealyticum*
    b. is a universally recognised cause of non-gonococcal urethritis
    c. is a well-recognised cause of Reiter's syndrome
    d. can cause pelvic inflammatory disease
    e. is usually eradicated by tetracyclines

For answers see over

Answers

A.9.12   a. F

           b. F—The role of *M. hominis* in the development of NGU is still unclear.

           c. F

           d. T

           e. T—Tetracyclines are the drugs of first choice for infections with *M. hominis*.

10. *Bacterial Vaginosis, Candidiasis and Trichomoniasis*

Q.10.1 **Vaginal clue cells**

a. indicate an underlying gonococcal infection
b. are epithelial cells coated with candidal spores
c. are never present in the normal vagina
d. support the diagnosis of bacterial vaginosis
e. are best visualised by phase contrast or dark-ground illumination

Q.10.2 **Bacterial vaginosis**

a. is associated with an overgrowth of *Gardnerella vaginalis* in the vagina
b. does not occur after the menopause
c. has been associated with the development of postpartum endometritis
d. is strongly associated with the development of cervical intraepithelial neoplasia
e. is associated with a decrease in the vaginal fluid amine content

Q.10.3 **A diagnosis of bacterial vaginosis is supported by the presence of**

a. a thin homogenous discharge
b. the presence of clue cells on microscopy of a Gram stained vaginal smear
c. a positive amine test on addition of dilute hydrochloric acid to the vaginal discharge
d. a vaginal pH of less than 4.5
e. marked vulval erythema

Q.10.4 **Bacterial vaginosis may be effectively treated with**

a. oxytetracycline
b. metronidazole
c. clotrimazole pessaries
d. fluconazole
e. povidone–iodine pessaries

For answers see over

Answers

A.10.1   a.   F—They give a 'clue' to the presence of bacterial vaginosis.
          b.   F—They are epithelial cells coated by coccobacilli.
          c.   F—They may be present in about 40% of women without bacterial vaginosis.
          d.   T
          e.   T—Using a wet preparation of vaginal discharge. Gram staining is also useful.

A.10.2   a.   T—It is due to an overgrowth of *Gardnerella vaginalis*, *Bacteroides* spp. and *Mobiluncus* spp.
          b.   F—It may occur at any age, although the maximum incidence is during the period of maximum sexual activity.
          c.   T
          d.   F
          e.   F—It is associated with an increase in amines such as putrescine and cadaverine, which are responsible for the fishy odour of the discharge.

A.10.3   a.   T
          b.   T
          c.   F—10% potassium hydroxide is added with characteristic enhancement of the fishy odour.
          d.   F
          e.   F—Three of the following four criteria are required to support a diagnosis of bacterial vaginosis:
               1   A vaginal pH > 4.5
               2   A fishy smelling discharge
               3   The presence of clue cells on a wet preparation
               4   A thin homogenous discharge.

A.10.4   a.   F
          b.   T—This is the treatment of choice, with a regimen of 500 mg twice daily for one week being effective. Relapse rates of 14%–40% have been described.
          c.   T—These may be effective and can be used during pregnancy.
          d.   F
          e.   T

Q.10.5   Candidal infection of the vagina

    a. causes a thick curdy vaginal discharge

    b. if asymptomatic requires treatment

    c. is associated with a vaginal pH of greater than 5

    d. may cause superficial dyspareunia

    e. is due to *Candida glabrata* in approximately 40% of cases

Q.10.6   The following agents commonly cause a vaginitis

    a. *Candida albicans*

    b. *Mycoplasma hominis*

    c. *Gardnerella vaginalis*

    d. *Trichomonas vaginalis*

    e. *Neisseria gonorrhoeae*

Q.10.7   The following conditions predispose to candidal infection:

    a. Pregnancy

    b. Hypertension

    c. Diabetes insipidus

    d. Antibiotic therapy

    e. Hypoparathyroidism

Q.10.8   *Trichomonas vaginalis* infection in women

    a. is associated with concurrent gonorrhoea in up to 40% of cases

    b. may cause punctate bleeding of the vaginal wall

    c. is associated with an alkaline pH of the vaginal fluid

    d. is always transmitted sexually

    e. is asymptomatic in up to 80% of cases

For answers see over

Answers

A.10.5 a. T
        b. F—It may occur in 40%–60% of women without causing symptoms.
        c. F
        d. T—Due to vulvitis and vaginitis.
        e. F—*Candida glabrata* is responsible for 10%–20% of cases of candidal vaginitis. It may be more difficult to treat due to resistance to imidazoles.

A.10.6 a. T
        b. F
        c. F—This causes a vaginosis – inflammatory cells are uncommon.
        d. T
        e. F—Although it may cause a vulvo-vaginitis in prepubescent females.

A.10.7 a. T
        b. F
        c. F—Diabetes mellitus predisposes to vaginal candidosis and also to balanitis.
        d. T—Although there is some debate as to the validity of this.
        e. T—This may be associated with chronic mucocutaneous infection.

A.10.8 a. T—This is a well-described association in sexually transmitted disease clinic attenders.
        b. T—This is more often seen on the cervix where it is described as 'strawberry' cervix.
        c. T
        d. F—It is thought that transmission via fomites, contaminated baths etc., may occasionally be responsible. Transmission from mother to baby may also occur.
        e. F—Approximately 40% of women do not complain of discharge.

Q.10.9 **The following infectious agents are correctly matched with their associated conditions:**

    a. *Gardnerella vaginalis* – bacterial vaginosis
    b. *Candida albicans* – strawberry cervix
    c. *Trichomonas vaginalis* – pelvic inflammatory disease
    d. *Neisseria gonorrhoeae* – Bartholin's abscess
    e. Bacteroides species and peptostreptococci – bacterial vaginosis

Q.10.10 *Trichomonas vaginalis*

    a. is a Gram positive bacterium
    b. may cause urethritis in the male
    c. leads to a yellow frothy irritating vaginal discharge
    d. may be cultured on Feinberg—Whittington medium
    e. is best diagnosed by Gram-stained smear from the lateral vaginal wall

Q.10.11 *Trichomonas vaginalis* **may be adequately treated by**

    a. Metronidazole
    b. Tinidazole
    c. Metformin
    d. Erythromycin
    e. Ciprofloxacin

Q.10.12 **The following infectious agents give a specific appearance on a Papanicolaou smear:**

    a. *Candida albicans*
    b. *Neisseria gonorrhoeae*
    c. *Gardnerella vaginalis*
    d. *Trichomonas vaginalis*
    e. Actinomycosis

For answers see over

Answers

A.10.9 a. T
        b. F—This is seen with *Trichomonas vaginalis*.
        c. T—The carriage of organisms such as *Neisseria gonorrhoeae* and *Chlamydia trachomatis* by *Trichomonas vaginalis* to the upper genital tract has been hypothesised.
        d. T
        e. T

A.10.10 a. F—It is a flagellate protozoan.
        b. T—Although it accounts for less than 1% of non-gonococcal urethritis in Great Britain.
        c. T—It may also lead to severe vulvitis.
        d. T—This contains liver digest, serum, antifungal and antibacterial agents.
        e. F—Secretions from the posterior fornix are best examined. Lateral wall vaginal sampling is the site of choice for the diagnosis of candidal infection.

A.10.11 a. T—Either a single dose of 2 g, or a week's course of 400 mg twice daily is recommended.
        b. T
        c. F
        d. F
        e. F

A.10.12 a. T
        b. F
        c. F
        d. T
        e. T—Herpes simplex virus and human papilloma virus infection may also be diagnosed on a Papanicolaou smear.

11. *Pelvic Inflammatory Disease, Family Planning, Ectopics*

Q.11.1 **The following conditions are included in the definition of pelvic inflammatory disease (PID):**

a. Pelvic peritonitis
b. Salpingo-oophoritis
c. Cervicitis
d. Endometritis
e. Urethritis

Q.11.2 **The long-term sequelae of PID include:**

a. Chronic pelvic pain
b. Tubal infertility
c. Recurrent early pregnancy loss
d. Increased risk of ectopic pregnancy
e. Anovulatory cycles

Q.11.3 **In a patient with lower abdominal pain, clinical features which support a diagnosis of PID are**

a. pyrexia
b. unilateral lower abdominal pain
c. haemoglobin less than 10 g/litre
d. serum ß-human chorionic gonadotrophin (HCG) greater than 400 units
e. purulent cervical discharge

Q.11.4 **Answer true or false:**

a. PID is usually sexually acquired
b. Eighty per cent of women with gonorrhoea develop salpingitis
c. Penicillin and metronidazole are adequate for the treatment of most cases of PID
d. Bed rest and attention to general health is important in the management of PID
e. Pelvic inflammatory disease is rare in pregnancy

For answers see over

Answers

A.11.1 a. T
  b. T
  c. F
  d. T
  e. F
  The term PID is normally used to describe infection of the upper female genital tract. The division between the upper and lower genital tracts is the cervix; therefore any infection at or below the cervix is a lower genital tract infection.

A.11.2 a. T
  b. T
  c. F
  d. T
  e. F
  Infertility after PID is due to tubal damage, which in turn leads to an increased risk of ectopic pregnancy. The menstrual cycle is not affected and the cause of recurrent early pregnancy loss has yet to be established, although postendometritis intrauterine adhesions have been suggested.

A.11.3 a. T—Fever may occur but is less pronounced in ectopic pregnancy or painful ovarian cysts.
  b. F—More common with an ectopic pregnancy.
  c. F—See answer b.
  d. F—See answer b.
  e. T—PID may also occur without any cervical discharge.

A.11.4 a. T—The most common agents causing PID are sexually transmitted – *Chlamydia trachomatis* and *Neisseria gonorrhoeae*. PID is very rare in women who are not sexually active.
  b. F—Only 10% of women with cervical gonorrhoea develop ascending infection.
  c. F—Penicillin and metronidazole would probably successfully treat many cases due to gonorrhoea and anaerobic bacteria but this regimen does not cover *Chlamydia trachomatis*.
  d. T
  e. T

Q.11.5 **Agents known to be responsible for acute salpingitis are**

a. *T. vaginalis*
b. *G. vaginalis*
c. *E. coli*
d. Staphylococci
e. *C. trachomatis*

Q.11.6 **Factors predisposing to an increased risk of acquiring acute salpingitis include**

a. use of the oral contraceptive pill
b. frequent change of sexual partners
c. previous episode of bacterial vaginosis
d. previous tubal surgery
e. age greater than 35 years

Q.11.7 **Barriers to the upward spread of infection from the cervix include**

a. the small diameter of the cervical canal
b. the upward flow of cervical mucus
c. the presence within mucus of lysozyme
d. the presence of secretory IgD in the mucus
e. are enhanced during pregnancy

Q.11.8 **Laparoscopy is indicated in the investigation of suspected PID in**

a. severely ill patients with suspected septicaemia
b. virgins
c. women aged over 45 years
d. women with a history of menstrual irregularity
e. if no therapeutic response is seen after 48–72 hours of antibiotic therapy

For answers see over

Answers

A.11.5   a. F
           b. F
           c. T
           d. T
           e. T

A.11.6   a. F—The oral contraceptive is thought to be protective.
           b. T
           c. F—Previous episodes of bacterial vaginosis are not relevant.
           d. T—It is thought that damaged Fallopian tubes are more easily infected.
           e. F—The age range of greatest incidence is 20–24 years.

A.11.7   a. T
           b. F—This is a downward flow.
           c. T—Lysozyme is an enzyme capable of hydrolysing peptidoglycan linkages in bacterial cell walls.
           d. F—IgA which is thought to be most important.
           e. T—This accounts for why PID is rare in pregnancy.

A.11.8   a. T
           b. T
           c. T—As the possibility of malignancy increases with age.
           d. T—This symptom increases the likelihood of ectopic pregnancy.
           e. T

Q.11.9 **Perihepatitis (Fitz Hugh Curtis syndrome)**

    a. occurs in about 4% of cases of acute pelvic inflammatory disease

    b. is commonly due to infection from the pelvis spreading via the right paracolic gutter

    c. is characterised by the formation of violin string adhesions between the liver and the stomach

    d. produces symptoms of upper abdominal pain and occasionally shoulder tip pain

    e. may undergo malignant change

Q.11.10 **The effective use of condoms by a male to prevent pregnancy**

    a. also provides 100% protection against sexually transmitted infections

    b. results in a failure rate of less than 0.7 per hundred couple years

    c. is enhanced by the use of spermicide

    d. is reduced by the use of oil-based lubricants such as vaseline

    e. may be supplemented by postcoital contraception if the condom breaks

Q.11.11 **The use of the combined oral contraceptive pill**

    a. has a pregnancy failure rate of only 3 per hundred woman years

    b. is contraindicated in women with crescendo migraine

    c. is contraindicated in Gilbert's disease

    d. is contraindicated with a recent history of trophoblastic disease

    e. is contraindicated in women with a history of cholestatic jaundice of pregnancy

Q.11.12 **The following are relative contraindications to the use of the combined oral contraceptive pill:**

    a. Crohn's disease

    b. Hyperprolactinaemia

    c. Sickle cell trait

    d. A past history of premalignant epithelial atypia in a breast biopsy

    e. Asthma

For answers see over

Answers

A.11.9 a. T
b. T—Lymphatic spread has also been hypothesised.
c. F—These adhesions are seen between the liver and the peritoneum.
d. T—Diaphragmatic irritation can lead to shoulder tip pain.
e. F

A.11.10 a. F—Condoms are impermeable to the causative agents of most sexually transmitted diseases. However, leakage of secretions and infectious agents spread by other sexual contact means that they do not confer 100% protection. Furthermore, non-penile infections may occur with agents such as scabies, crabs, HSV and HPV.
b. T—With lower rates being observed in more experienced condom-using couples.
c. T
d. T
e. T

A.11.11 a. F—The rate is 0.2–0.5 per hundred woman years.
b. T
c. F
d. T
e. T

A.11.12 a. T
b. T
c. F
d. T
e. F

Q.11.13 The following reduce the effectiveness of concurrently administered oral contraceptive pills:

a. Ampicillin
b. Cotrimoxazole
c. Tetracycline
d. Rifampicin
e. Griseofulvin

Q.11.14 In a woman using an intrauterine contraceptive device (IUCD) the following features increase her risk of developing PID:

a. Younger age
b. Previous history of sexually transmitted infection
c. Use of a monofilament design
d. Oestrogen implanted devices
e. Recent insertion of the IUCD

Q.11.15 Postcoital contraception can be effectively provided by the following methods:

a. The Yuzpe method within five days
b. The provision of two tablets containing 250 MCG of levonorgestrol with 50 MCG of ethinyloestradiol given at once followed by a further two tablets twelve hours later
c. Insertion of a copper-bearing intrauterine device
d. 2 mg of vinblastine given intramuscularly stat
e. Ethinyloestrodiol within 72 hours of a single exposure

Q.11.16 Answer true or false to the following statements about postcoital contraception:

a. Follow-up is not essential providing a woman reassures you that she will use proper contraception next time
b. After the Yuzpe regimen the next period is usually on time
c. If a woman vomits the tablets prescribed for postcoital contraception, she must return to see her doctor immediately
d. If postcoital contraception with combined pills fails, it is mandatory for a woman to have an abortion
e. The history of a previous ectopic pregnancy is a relative contraindication to postcoital contraception

For answers see over

Answers

A.11.13 a. T
b. F
c. T
d. T
e. T

A.11.14 a. T
b. T
c. F—The Dalcon shield with its multifilament thread was shown to act as a wick for invading micro-organisms.
d. F—There has been suggestion that the use of progesterones in the IUCD may reduce the risk of infection, but this is unproven.
e. T

A.11.15 a. F
b. T—This is the Yuzpe method and should be given within 72 hours of unprotected intercourse.
c. T—This should be done not more than 5 days after the calculated date of ovulation.
d. F
e. T

A.11.16 a. F—Defined follow-up is vital and is normally set for 3–4 weeks post treatment.
b. F—It will be up to a week late or more in at least half of the women.
c. T—It may be important to consider inserting an IUCD or to provide additional tablets.
d. F—There is no evidence that the treatment will significantly increase the risk of fetal abnormalities.
e. T

Q.11.17 Ectopic pregnancy

a. is defined as the implantation of a conceptus outside the uterine cavity
b. occurs in the Fallopian tubes in 45% of cases
c. is initially incorrectly diagnosed in up to 50% of cases
d. has doubled in incidence in the UK over the past 20 years
e. produces signs of shock in patients at presentation in 75% of cases

Q.11.18 Predisposing factors which increase the likelihood of a pregnancy being situated in an extrauterine site are

a. previous history of pelvic inflammatory disease
b. previous tubal surgery
c. female sterilisation by tubal ligation
d. the use of an IUCD
e. the use of the combined oral contraceptive pill

Q.11.19 The clinical presentation of a woman with an ectopic pregnancy

a. will include a history of amenorrhoea in 95% of cases
b. may include vaginal bleeding with the passage of a decidual cast
c. includes an adnexal mass which is indicative of the site of the pregnancy in 75% of the cases
d. will feature the co-existence of an intrauterine and ectopic pregnancy in 1 in 5000 cases
e. is confirmed by a positive test for ßHCG in more than 95% of cases

Q.11.20 The management of a woman with a suspected ectopic pregnancy should include

a. an urgent full blood count
b. cross-matched blood available
c. an urgent ultrasound scan
d. immediate antibiotic prophylaxis with oral erythromycin and metronidazole
e. an urgent serum α-fetoprotein performed

For answers see over

Answers

A.11.17 a. T
         b. F—95% of cases occur in the Fallopian tubes.
         c. T
         d. T
         e. F—The figure is between 15% and 25%.

A.11.18 a. T—Evidence suggests that one previous episode of PID increases the risk of ectopic pregnancy ten fold.
         b. T
         c. T—This procedure decreases the incidence of pregnancy overall, but increases the ratio of ectopic to intrauterine pregnancy if a pregnancy does occur.
         d. T—Although this decreases the overall incidence of ectopic pregnancy it increases the ratio by ten fold of ectopic to intrauterine pregnancies if a pregnancy occurs.
         e. F—Progesterone-only pills do increase the likelihood that a pregnancy occurring on treatment will be ectopic.

A.11.19 a. F—Amenorrhoea occurs in approximately 75% of cases.
         b. T
         c. F—In half of these the pregnancy will be on the opposite side to that which the mass has been felt.
         d. F—The true rate is 1 in 30 000 cases except in cases of assisted conception where this is more common.
         e. T

A.11.20 a. T
         b. T
         c. T
         d. F—Unless local or systemic infection is strongly suspected, there is no evidence that antibiotics are necessary. Oral therapy should not be given as patients with suspected ectopics should be fasted until the diagnosis is established.
         e. F—Urgent serum ßHCG should be estimated

Q.11.21 **In a patient with suspected ectopic pregnancy immediate surgical intervention**

  a. should be delayed until an intravenous line is established and resuscitation of the shocked patient has been completed
  b. by laparoscopy is indicated in all women who present with painful vaginal bleeding, a positive pregnancy test and no intrauterine pregnancy visible on ultrasound scan
  c. should aim to perform salpingectomy as the operation of choice
  d. should be preceded by hysteroscopy to search for an intrauterine pregnancy in difficult cases
  e. By urgent laparoscopy is indicated in women who present with shock

For answers see over

Answers

A.11.21 a. F—Immediate surgery to prevent continued haemorrhage is essential if resuscitation is to be efficacious and thus should not be delayed by attempts at resuscitation. Rather the two should occur contemporaneously.

b. T

c. F—Salpingectomy should be avoided if possible. However, haemostasis is the priority for all cases.

d. F

e. F—Immediate laparotomy is essential in such cases.

12. *Colposcopy*

Q.12.1 **A clear epidemiological association with cervical cancer has been shown for women**

a. with a past history of gonorrhoea
b. with genital warts
c. who are cigarette smokers
d. with a past history of herpes genitalis
e. who have used oral contraceptives

Q.12.2 **No association with an increased risk of developing cervical intraepithelial neoplasia (CIN) has been shown for**

a. multiple sexual partners
b. early age of first intercourse
c. using an intrauterine contraceptive device
d. repeated episodes of bacterial vaginosis
e. oral herpes simplex infection

Q.12.3 **Probable causes of an increased number of polymorpho-nuclear cells in the cervix include**

a. oral contraceptive use
b. human papillomavirus infection
c. gonorrhoea
d. *Chlamydia trachomatis*
e. acquiring a new sexual partner

Q.12.4 **The following groups of women should be targetted for more frequent cytological screening:**

a. Prostitutes
b. Women with genital warts
c. Women with immunosuppression
d. Women with recurrent bacterial vaginosis
e. Women whose regular sexual partner has genital warts

For answers see over

Answers

A.12.1 a. T—Furgyk and Asted in 1980 demonstrated an association but did not test whether this was causal.

           b. T

           c. T

           d. T

           e. F—No clear association has been shown. Studies are confounded by contraceptive use being influenced by patterns of sexual behaviour.

A.12.2 a. F

           b. F

           c. T

           d. T

           e. T

A.12.3 a. T—This is an effect of progesterone dominance.

           b. F

           c. T

           d. T

           e. T—Especially in younger women, a strong inflammatory response to foreign sperm and seminal fluid may be found which is thought to be a normal reaction.

A.12.4 a. T

           b. T

           c. T

           d. F

           e. T

Recent studies suggest that women in the above risk groups should have annual cytological (and possibly colposcopic) examination of their cervix. However, as yet limited resources and unclear benefits confine this service to research projects.

Q.12.5 **Colposcopy is best performed**

    a. on or about day 2 of the menstrual cycle
    b. before taking a routine cervical smear
    c. at mid-cycle
    d. with the patient under a general anaesthetic
    e. with the aim of obtaining directed biopsies for histological diagnosis

Q.12.6 **Cytological examination of a Papanicolaou cervical smear has a high specificity in diagnosing the following conditions:**

    a. Bacterial vaginosis
    b. Gonorrhoea
    c. Herpes simplex virus infection
    d. Human papillomavirus infection
    e. Actinomycosis

Q.12.7 **Cervical columnar epithelium**

    a. is ten cells thick
    b. does not produce mucus
    c. stains dark brown after application of Lugol's iodine
    d. has a typical 'cluster of grapes' appearance
    e. always lines the entire endocervical canal

For answers see over

Answers

A.12.5   a. F—Colposcopy is difficult during menstruation as blood may occlude full vision.
b. F—Colposcopy is not designed to replace cytological screening. The effects of acetic acid on the subsequent smear may affect the cellular appearance.
c. T—This is the ideal time to perform colposcopy, as the external os is wide open and the mucus is clear.
d. F
e. T—In addition to identifying the extent of the abnormal epithelium, this is the main aim of the colposcopist.

A.12.6   a. F
b. F
c. T—Large multinucleate giant cells reliably diagnose HSV infections.
d. T—Koilocytes (vacuolated epithelial cells) are indicative of wart virus (HPV) infection.
e. F
a, b and e cannot reliably be diagnosed on a Papanicolaou smear. c and d do not have a high sensitivity, but are highly specific for their respective infections if found.

A.12.7   a. F—It is one cell thick. Squamous epithelium is 15–20 cells thick.
b. F—Columnar epithelium produces mucus.
c. F—Columnar epithelium does not take up the iodine stain as it does not contain glycogen, squamous epithelium does.
d. T—The glandular mucosa is not smooth. It covers numerous connective tissue papillae, thus giving an appearance of numerous minute polyps.
e. F—The squamocolumnar junction can lie in the cervical canal, and therefore some squamous epithelium can line the lower end of the canal. This occurs after the menopause or following local destructive therapy (e.g. cone biopsy or diathermy).

Q.12.8 The squamocolumnar junction (SCJ) of the cervix:

a. is always visible at colposcopy
b. is a junction between a 16-cell-thick and a 1-cell-thick epithelium
c. becomes more ectocervical after the menopause
d. becomes endocervical with the use of oestrogens
e. is the only site of Nabothian follicles

Q.12.9 The following are features of an atypical transformation zone on the cervix:

a. Whitening after application of acetic acid
b. Lack of mosaic pattern
c. Punctuation pattern
d. Nabothian follicles
e. Complete uptake of Lugol's iodine

Q.12.10 Colposcopy

a. was initiated in 1924 by Hinselman who designed a low power microscope with which he expected to see early 'mini-cancers'
b. is contraindicated in a woman with a coagulation disorder
c. should include an inspection of the vagina and vulva as well as the cervix
d. often involves the application of 20% acetic acid to the cervix
e. with Monsell's solution is used to demonstrate healthy mature glycogenated squamous epithelium

For answers see over

Answers

A.12.8 a. F—The site of the SCJ is variable and therefore not always visible if situated within the endocervical canal.
   b. T
   c. F—After the menopause, due to lack of oestrogens, the cervix atrophies and involutes. Thus the SCJ recedes up the canal.
   d. F—The SCJ becomes more ectocervical (also at puberty and during pregnancy).
   e. F—Nabothian follicles arise in the columnar epithelium and are therefore also found in the transformation zone, not just along the SCJ.

A.12.9 a. T—This is the typical reaction of abnormal epithelium.
   b. F—Lack of mosaic pattern is the appearance of a typical transformation zone.
   c. T—Both the mosaic and punctuation patterns represent abnormal vascular patterns, indicating the need for a biopsy to make a diagnosis.
   d. F—These are features of a normal transformation zone.
   e. F—The reverse is true. Abnormal squamous epithelium does not contain glycogen, and therefore fails to take up the stain.

A.12.10 a. T—But his aim was not fulfilled although he was able to describe definitive patterns suggestive of premalignant disease.
   b. F—Colposcopy itself is not contraindicated, but care should be taken when taking cervical biopsies.
   c. T
   d. F—3%–5% acetic acid is normally used. Higher strengths may cause severe local chemical irritation.
   e. F—Schiller's or Lugol's iodine is used for this purpose. Monsell's solution (ferric subsulphate) is a styptic compound which is often used to assist haemostasis after biopsy.

Q.12.11 **Prior to performing local ablative therapy for CIN lesions the colposcopist should be confident that**

a. the atypical transformation zone does not reveal any suggestion of invasive cancer
b. the colposcopy examination should reveal more than 50% of any intracervical lesion
c. histological evidence of microinvasion is to a depth of less than 8 mm
d. endometrial curettings are negative for any evidence of dysplasia
e. at least three consecutive cervical smears have confirmed evidence of dyskaryosis

Q.12.12 **Acceptable modalities for local destructive treatments of CIN are**

a. cryotherapy
b. cold coagulation
c. electrodiathermy
d. carbon dioxide laser vaporisation
e. suction curettage

Q.12.13 **Excisional techniques for the treatment of CIN include**

a. cold knife biopsy
b. large-loop diathermy
c. laser conisation
d. hysterectomy
e. laser hysteroscopy

Q.12.14 **Large-loop excision of the transformation zone (LLETZ)**

a. was first described by Cartier as a technique for improving the size of samples taken by punch biopsies
b. for treatment of CIN takes between 20 and 25 minutes in 90% of cases
c. is accompanied by a 15% risk of secondary haemorrhage
d. always requires general anaesthetic
e. provides a sample for histopathological examination in 75% of cases

For answers see over

Answers

A.12.11 a. T
  b. F—For a colposcopy to be deemed satisfactory it is vital that no endocervical extension of lesions is outside of the operator's vision.
  c. F—This cannot be assessed by colposcopy, only by the histopathologist looking at a biopsy.
  d. F
  e. F

A.12.12 a. T
  b. T
  c. T
  d. T
  e. F

A.12.13 a. T
  b. T
  c. T
  d. T—This is usually indicated for women with another strong indication for hysterectomy (eg. fibroids), or women who have had repeated recurrences of CIN after multiple local excisional procedures.
  e. F

A.12.14 a. T
  b. F—In one study the mean time for duration of this treatment was 3.47 minutes.
  c. F—Primary or secondary bleeding complications are rare with this type of therapy.
  d. F—LLETZ can be performed without anaesthetic but most operators make use of local anaesthetic and haemostatic injections prior to therapy.
  e. F—This technique produces a sample for analysis to confirm the grade of abnormality present and the extent of clearance at the margins.

Q.12.15 **The management of an abnormal Papanicolaou smear in a pregnant woman**

    a. is termination of pregnancy for CIN III lesions

    b. includes standard colposcopic assessment

    c. is complicated by cervical eversion

    d. should be conservative unless there is any suggestion of invasion

    e. should not include cervical biopsy as this may lead to premature labour

Q.12.16 **Follow-up of women treated for CIN lesions by local therapy should**

    a. include cytology and colposcopy

    b. Be aimed at detecting recurrences occurring between 5 and 10 years later

    c. Be at more frequent intervals for women with HPV 16 or 18 infection

    d. include the use of an endocervical brush to sample the endocervix in all cases

    e. include cytology and colposcopy follow-up for at least five years

Q.12.17 **Glandular dysplasia of the cervix**

    a. is more common than squamous dysplasia

    b. has an intraepithelial stage called adeno-carcinoma in situ

    c. is preinvasive in most cases of detected disease

    d. is poorly diagnosed by colposcopy or cytology

    e. is best treated by excisional rather than ablative therapy

For answers see over

Answers

A.12.15 a. F
        b. T
        c. F—Pregnancy, by causing cervical eversion, facilitates visualisation of the transformation zone.
        d. T
        e. F—Although this should only be performed if a progressive or high-grade lesion is suspected.

A.12.16 a. T
        b. F—The commonest recurrences seem to be in the first or second year after therapy.
        c. F—There are no data to suggest that the detection of any particular HPV type should be managed by more frequent follow-up visits.
        d. F—Although this is useful in women in whom the transformation zone extends into the cervical canal.
        e. F—Most units have rationalised the facility for cytological and colposcopy follow-up to the first two years after therapy. Surveillance after this time is normally by repeat cytological screening at regular intervals.

A.12.17 a. F
        b. T
        c. F
        d. T
        e. T—Care in ensuring adequate margins of excision are vital in planning follow-up.

13. *STDs in Pregnancy*

Q.13.1 **Concerning syphilis in pregnancy:**

a. A positive VDRL of 1/8 with a negative TPHA requires treatment with penicillin
b. In penicillin-allergic patients, oxytetracycline is the treatment of choice
c. Women with previously treated syphilis and a positive TPHA in early pregnancy need to be retreated
d. Infection may lead to mid-trimester abortion
e. Infants of mothers with latent syphilis may be born with congenital syphilis

Q.13.2 **Genital herpes infection during pregnancy**

a. is associated with fetal eighth nerve damage
b. is best managed with suppressive doses of acyclovir in the first trimester
c. should never be treated with acyclovir
d. may lead to disseminated disease in the neonate
e. may be associated with spontaneous abortion

Q.13.3 **Genital warts during pregnancy**

a. are safely treated with 10% but not 25% podophyllin
b. may become unresponsive to treatment
c. may enlarge considerably and cause obstruction to labour
d. may be confused with condylomata lata
e. may result in laryngeal papillomata in the neonate

For answers see over

Answers

A.13.1 a. F—This may represent a biological false positive reaction and should be monitored by repeat serology and clinical examination to exclude the possibility of early syphilis.

b. F—This is contraindicated due to the effects on growing bone and dentition. Erythromycin is the treatment of choice, but due to poor placental transfer some advocate full penicillin treatment of the neonate.

c. F—The 'specific' treponemal tests, ie. the FTA and TPHA typically remain positive following treatment. However, some centres advocate retreatment as a 'failsafe'.

d. T

e. T—Although patients with late latent syphilis are unlikely to transmit the disease sexually, it may be transmitted transplacentally.

A.13.2 a. F

b. F—Acyclovir is not licensed for use during pregnancy as there is inadequate evidence as to safety.

c. F—In severe genital herpes or disseminated disease, acyclovir should be considered.

d. T

e. T—Particularly with severe primary genital herpes.

A.13.3 a. F—Podophyllin is contraindicated in pregnancy, due to its potential teratogenic effect.

b. T—The physiological 'immunosuppression' which accompanies pregnancy may lead to the warts becoming recalcitrant.

c. T—Bushke Löwenstein tumour must be considered.

d. T—The condylomata lata of secondary syphilis may appear similar to condylomata acuminata.

e. T

Q.13.4 **Concerning urinary tract infection in pregnancy:**

a. If recurrent, it requires investigation in the puerperium
b. Is best treated by cotrimoxazole if due to *Escherichia coli*
c. Ureteric dilatation due to maternal oestrogens predisposes to infection
d. If it is asymptomatic, it does not need treatment
e. Requires intravenous therapy if dysuria and frequency are present

Q.13.5 **Answer true or false to the following:**

a. Maternal *Candida albicans* infection must be treated during pregnancy
b. Metronidazole may be safely used to treat *Trichomonas* infection in the third trimester
c. Chlamydial ophthalmia neonatorum usually presents within two days of birth
d. Maternal chlamydial infection may lead to pneumonitis in the neonate
e. Ciprofloxacin 500 mg as a single dose is the treatment of choice for uncomplicated genital gonorrhoea in pregnant women

Q.13.6 **Caesarean section is indicated**

a. in women with extensive genital warts occluding the vagina
b. in women with a history of recurrent genital herpes
c. in women with a primary chancre of the vulva
d. in women with CIN
e. in women with HIV infection

For answers see over

Answers

A.13.4 a. T—Intravenous urography (IVU) supplemented by cystoscopy is indicated to exclude any structural abnormalities. Some centres would now use ultrasound instead of IVU.

      b. F—Cotrimoxazole should be avoided during pregnancy. Ampicillin or nitrofurantoin would be the treatment of choice.

      c. F—Ureteric dilation leading to stasis is thought to occur due to progesterone.

      d. F—The risk of pyelonephritis necessitates treatment.

      e. F—Oral therapy is adequate unless there is evidence of pyelonephritis.

A.13.5 a. F—As in the non-pregnant state, asymptomatic candida does not require treatment.

      b. T

      c. F—The incubation period is 3–13 days. Gonococcal ophthalmia normally presents within the first 48 hours.

      d. T

      e. F—Ciprofloxacin should be avoided because of a potential adverse effect on developing cartilage. Spectinomycin may be used.

A.13.6 a. T—There may be mechanical obstruction of the labour canal.

      b. F—Some centres advocate Caesarean section in the presence of visible vulval or cervical ulcers, if the membranes have not ruptured.

      c. F—Syphilis is a systemic disease from the outset and this will not necessarily prevent neonatal infection.

      d. F

      e. F—Although some data suggest that, in some cases, this may reduce vertical transmission of HIV during labour.

14. *Dermatoses and Infestations*

Q.14.1 Lichen sclerosus (LS)

a. only occurs in males
b. never occurs before puberty
c. responds well to hydrocortisone-containing creams
d. never undergoes malignant transformation
e. characteristically shows elongated rete ridges on histology

Q.14.2 Circinate balanitis

a. is always associated with concurrent chlamydial urethritis
b. is histologically identical to psoriasis
c. is best treated with local antibacterial creams
d. occasionally undergoes malignant transformation
e. characteristically has a spontaneously relapsing and remitting course

Q.14.3 Buschke—Löwenstein tumours

a. are associated with infection by HPV 16
b. frequently metastasise
c. may be locally invasive
d. are usually treated by systemic chemotherapy
e. only occur in the anogenital area

Q.14.4 Bowenoid papulosis:

a. Is another name for Bowen's disease
b. Is usually associated with infection with HPV type 16
c. Is rarely pigmented
d. Is a form of intraepithelial neoplasia
e. May occur outside the anogenital area

Q.14.5 Erythrasma

a. is caused by group B streptococci
b. typically causes well-outlined, dry patches covered with fine desquamation in the genitocrural folds
c. is frequently very itchy
d. is best diagnosed by Gram staining of scrapings from the lesion sites
e. is best treated by topical imidazole creams

For answers see over

Answers

A.14.1 a. F—The reported incidence is higher in women than in men.
           b. F
           c. F—However, higher potency steroid creams may be of use.
           d. F—The malignant potential of LS is currently unclear, although probably very low.
           e. F—This is a feature of psoriasis. LS shows marked hyperkeratosis in association with severe epidermal atrophy.

A.14.2 a. F—It can occur with other causes of Reiter's syndrome.
           b. T
           c. F—Simple reassurance is usually effective. Steroid creams may be helpful.
           d. F
           e. T

A.14.3 a. F—HPV 6 is most commonly found.
           b. F—The tumours rarely become malignant.
           c. T
           d. F—Local treatment is usually adequate.
           e. F—Extragenital lesions have been rarely reported.

A.14.4 a. F—Bowen's disease is a type of carcinoma *in situ*.
           b. T
           c. F
           d. T
           e. T

A.14.5 a. F—The causative agent is *Corynebacterium minutissimum*.
           b. T
           c. F
           d. T
           e. F—Systemic tetracyclines are the treatment of choice.

Q.14.6   Psoriasis

a. is associated with HLA types B13 and B17
b. may occur exclusively in the genital area
c. may be associated with Wickham's striae
d. when occurring in the genital area, is best treated with coal tar preparations
e. may show the Koebner phenomenon

Q.14.7   Lichen planus

a. tends to have a relapsing and remitting course
b. causes violaceous, pruritic papules
c. is best treated by radiotherapy
d. may be associated with hyperpigmentation and atrophy on healing
e. may be associated with nail changes

Q.14.8   Drug eruptions

a. of the Stevens–Johnson type may be fatal
b. may be the cause of genital ulceration
c. have characteristic histopathological features
d. are less common in HIV seropositive individuals as a result of their immunosuppression
e. never occur during the first course of any treatment

Q.14.9   Plasma cell balanitis

a. is associated with certain haematological malignancies
b. typically causes a moist, smooth patch of erythema in the preputial sac
c. is associated with a circulating lymphocytosis
d. is best treated with topical steroids
e. is regarded as a premalignant condition

For answers see over

Answers

A.14.6 a. T
        b. T
        c. F—Wickham's striae are associated with lichen planus.
        d. F—Coal tar is generally regarded as too irritant for the genital
            area. Reassurance of the patient alone may be adequate.
            Low potency steroid creams may be sparingly used.
        e. T

A.14.7 a. F—The majority of people have one episode, although
            recurrences occasionally occur.
        b. T
        c. F—Reassurance is usually adequate. Steroid creams with
            antipruritic medication may be of value in severe cases.
        d. T
        e. T

A.14.8 a. T
        b. T
        c. F—The diagnosis is usually made on clinical grounds.
        d. F
        e. F

A.14.9 a. F
        b. T
        c. F
        d. T
        e. F

Q.14.10 Behçet's syndrome

    a. only occurs in people of Japanese and eastern Mediterranean extraction
    b. may be spread by sexual contact
    c. is associated with recurrent genital and oral ulceration
    d. characteristically causes ulcers on the glans penis and labia
    e. responds to treatment with acyclovir

Q.14.11 Carcinoma of the penis

    a. accounts for between 5% and 10% of all male malignancies in Western Europe
    b. rarely occurs in those circumcised in the neonatal period
    c. is thought to occur more commonly in those with poor genital hygiene
    d. is more common in smokers
    e. is associated with HPV 16 and 18 in over 90% of cases

Q.14.12 Erythroplasia of Queyrat

    a. causes characteristic bowing of the erect penis
    b. is histologically indistinguishable from Bowen's disease
    c. predominantly affects men
    d. can usually be diagnosed on clinical appearance alone
    e. usually responds completely to topical hydrocortisone therapy

Q.14.13 *Phthirus pubis*

    a. is a louse
    b. lays its eggs in burrows
    c. lives off skin squames
    d. rarely survives off the host for more than 24 hours
    e. is invisible to the naked eye

Q.14.14 Crab louse infestation

    a. only occurs in the genital area
    b. can occasionally occur in dogs
    c. is always transmitted sexually
    d. may be asymptomatic
    e. is characteristically itchy

For answers see over

Answers

A.14.10 a. F—Although it is more common in these groups.
      b. F
      c. T
      d. T
      e. F

A.14.11 a. F—It is much rarer than this.
      b. T
      c. T
      d. F
      e. F—HPV 16 and 18 have been found in approximately 50% of lesions.

A.14.12 a. F—This is typically caused by Peyronie's disease.
      b. T
      c. T—Usually the foreskin and glans.
      d. F—Biopsy of suspect lesions is necessary.
      e. F—Excision, electron beam therapy or 5-fluorouracil are most likely to be effective.

A.14.13 a. T
      b. F—The eggs are attached to the bases of hairs.
      c. F—It is a blood-sucking parasite.
      d. T
      e. F—It can easily be seen by the unaided eye, moving about in the genital hair-bearing area.

A.14.14 a. F—It also occurs in other hair-bearing areas.
      b. T
      c. F—Occasional fomite transmission has been reported.
      d. T
      e. T

Q.14.15 In the diagnosis of crab louse infestation

a. the method of choice is to look for a fourfold rise in complement-fixing antibody titre
b. the organism is usually cultivated in rabbit genital preparations
c. skin biopsy is often useful
d. clinical observation is usually sufficient
e. it is unnecessary to examine areas above the neck

Q.14.16 In the management of crab louse infestation

a. recent asymptomatic sexual contacts do not need to be treated
b. 1% gamma benzene hexachloride (lindane) is recommended for the treatment of small children
c. pyrethrins are of established use
d. vaseline is of use in the treatment of eyelash involvement
e. all clothes and bed linen used in the previous two days must be washed in 1% lindane solution

Q.14.17 *Sarcoptes scabiei*

a. is easily visible to the unaided eye in infected individuals
b. is more frequent among black Americans than among white Americans
c. can be transmitted by fomites
d. characteristically causes severe nocturnal itch
e. are typically present in thousands in infected individuals

Q.14.18 Clinical scabies

a. frequently affects the interdigital clefts of the hands
b. characteristically causes ulceration of the glans penis
c. is associated with burrows which follow skin lines
d. may present with urticaria as its only sign
e. is exacerbated by the inadvertent use of topical steroid creams

For answers see over

Answers

A.14.15 a. F
   b. F
   c. F
   d. T
   e. F—Extragenital infestation may occur. It is also important to examine the patient for other sexually transmitted conditions.

A.14.16 a. F—All recent sexual contacts should be offered examination and epidemiological treatment.
   b. F
   c. T
   d. T
   e. F—Conventional hot-washing is adequate to destroy the lice.

A.14.17 a. F
   b. F—The converse is true.
   c. T
   d. T
   e. F—Only a few mites are normally present on each infected individual.

A.14.18 a. T—This is the classical location of scabies.
   b. F—Penile involvement is usually nodular.
   c. F—The burrows cross skin lines.
   d. T
   e. T

Q.14.19 Crusted (Norwegian) scabies

a. is highly infectious
b. is clinically similar to psoriasis
c. may be associated with dystrophy of the nails
d. is characteristically extremely itchy
e. tends to occur in immunocompromised individuals

Q.14.20 In typical scabies

a. the diagnosis must be made by performing a skin biopsy
b. the whole body should be treated
c. asymptomatic household members do not need treatment unless there has been recent sexual contact
d. the patient remains infectious until pruritis settles
e. patients should wash their hands thoroughly following application of the antiscabetic preparation

Q.14.21 Peyronie's disease

a. was described in 1743
b. is always associated with Dupuytren's contracture
c. is the result of the development of fibrous penile plaques which cause pain and deformity
d. can be cured by vitamin E taken orally
e. should be treated early by surgery

Q.14.22 Erosive balanitis may be caused by

a. trichomonal infection
b. Reiter's disease
c. Zoon's balanitis
d. Lichen nitidis
e. fixed drug eruptions

Q.14.23 Plasma cell balanitis

a. is sometimes called Zoon's balanitis
b. results in painful penile and preputial ulcers
c. is associated with a systemic lymphopenia
d. may be treated by topical steroids
e. commonly undergoes malignant change

For answers see over

Answers

A.14.19 a. T
        b. T
        c. T
        d. F
        e. T

A.14.20 a. F—Clinical suspicion and a therapeutic trial with an antiscabetic preparation are usually adequate.
        b. F—It is unnecessary to treat above the neck.
        c. F—All household members should be offered epidemiological treatment.
        d. F—Provided that directions are followed fully, infectivity ceases within 24 hours.
        e. F—This may lead to inadequately treated scabies of the hands and subsequent re-establishment of the infestation.

A.14.21 a. T—By De la Peyronie
        b. F—Although familial cases with both conditions do occur.
        c. T
        d. F
        e. F

A.14.22 a. T
        b. T
        c. T
        d. F
        e. T

A.14.23 a. T
        b. F—It typically causes a glistening erythematous reddish-brown lesion with an arcuate edge.
        c. F
        d. T
        e. F

Q.14.24 **The following may be cutaneous manifestations of sexually transmitted infections**

    a. Hirsutes papillaris penis
    b. Keratoderma blennorrhagica
    c. Fordyce spots
    d. Condylomata lata
    e. Fox–Fordyce disease

For answers see over

Answers

A.14.24 a. F—This is a normal variant found in 10% of men.
b. T—In Reiters syndrome.
c. F—These are ectopic sebaceous glands often situated on the submucosa of the prepuce or vulva.
d. T
e. F—This is a disorder of the apocrine glands which can produce marked vulval pruritis.

15. *Psychosexual Problems, Assault and Prostitution*

Q.15.1   Child sexual abuse

    a. is largely unreported
    b. can confidently be diagnosed following isolation of *N. gonorrhoeae* from a vaginal swab
    c. may result in transmission of HIV
    d. is highly likely to have occurred if molluscum contagiosum are found on the child
    e. is often perpetrated by a family member

Q.15.2   In the management of women alleging sexual assault

    a. screening for sexually transmitted pathogens must be delayed until two weeks after the event
    b. HIV testing is mandatory
    c. postcoital contraception should be considered up to 7 days after the assault
    d. vaccination against hepatitis B should be considered
    e. prophylactic antibiotics are not generally indicated

Q.15.3   During normal sexual stimulation of the male

    a. the wall of the scrotum becomes thinner
    b. the testes become elevated
    c. the testes enlarge in size
    d. erection of the penis results from parasympathetically induced arterial dilatation
    e. ejaculation always occurs prior to loss of erection

Q.15.4   The following drugs result in erections when injected intracavernosally:

    a. Phenoxybenzamine
    b. Clonidine
    c. Papaverine
    d. Imipramine
    e. Phentolamine

For answers see over

Answers

A.15.1 a. T

b. F—Although abuse should be seriously considered.

c. T—There has been at least one documented case.

d. F—Molluscum contagiosum is common in children and usually spreads through non-sexual contact.

e. T

A.15.2 a. F—An initial screen is helpful to exclude infection occurring prior to the event.

b. F—Although serum may be saved to permit subsequent analysis if after careful counselling, the patient requests this.

c. T—The oral contraceptive pill may be used up to 72 hours after unprotected intercourse. An intrauterine contraceptive device may be inserted up to 7 days post coitus, although ascending infection is a possible risk.

d. T

e. T—Although they may be given if the assailant was suspected of having a sexually transmitted disease.

A.15.3 a. F—It becomes thicker and tighter due to local venous congestion as well as contraction of the dartos muscle.

b. T—Due to retraction of the spermatic cords and contraction of the cremaster muscle.

c. T

d. T

e. F

A.15.4 a. T—The erection produced lasts up to six hours.

b. F—This causes shrinkage of erectile tissue.

c. T—Erections last between two and two and a half hours.

d. F—This causes shrinkage of erectile tissue.

e. T—This causes an erection lasting up to ten minutes only.

Q.15.5 Use of the following drugs has been associated with an increased incidence of erectile impotence:

    a. Guanethidine
    b. Indoramin
    c. Labetalol
    d. Diazepam
    e. Bendrofluazide

Q.15.6 Follow-up studies of patients who have undergone gender reassignment surgery in the treatment of transsexualism show that

    a. 50% of patients regret having the surgery after three years of follow-up
    b. female to male transsexuals achieve more social acceptance than do male to female transsexuals
    c. personal or social instability preoperatively is directly associated with an unsatisfactory postoperative outcome
    d. the older the age at which the reassignment is performed the better the outcome
    e. in male to female cases there is a high correlation between the sexual functioning of the surgically created vagina and the patient's satisfaction with the operation

Q.15.7 The following sexual problems are linked to their accompanying general medical conditions:

    a. Erectile dysfunction in men with diabetes mellitus
    b. Orgasmic dysfunction in women with diabetes mellitus
    c. Erectile and ejaculatory dysfunction and hypertension
    d. Reduction in sexual interest in both men and women with chronic renal failure
    e. Reduction in libido in both men and women with multiple sclerosis

For answers see over

Answers

A.15.5 a. T—This produced both erectile and ejaculatory dysfunction in more than 50% of patients receiving it.
 b. F—This alpha blocker has been reported to interfere with ejaculation in two-thirds of men taking it but to have no effect on erection.
 c. F—This alpha and beta blocking antihypertensive drug has been shown to lengthen the time which both male and female subjects take to reach orgasm but not to affect erection in male subjects.
 d. F—The use of this drug has been shown only to cause delayed orgasm in women.
 e. T

A.15.6 a. F—Only 5% regretted this.
 b. T
 c. T
 d. F
 e. T

A.15.7 a. T
 b. T—Whether this is due to an increase in vaginal infections, problems with lubrication, autonomic dysfunction or psychological problems, is not clear.
 c. T—It may be difficult to decide whether this is secondary to the disease or to treatment.
 d. T—For both psychological as well as metabollic and endocrine reasons.
 e. T

Q.15.8   **The following statements about female prostitutes are true:**

a. Controlled trials have demonstrated a high prevalence of hepatitis B infection among female prostitutes

b. Due to poor compliance with follow-up, longitudinal studies of sexually transmitted diseases among female prostitutes have not been able to be performed

c. Vaginal carriage of *M. hominis* and *Ureaplasma urealyticum* occurs in female prostitutes

d. The regular partners of female prostitutes are a major source of infection with sexually transmitted pathogens

e. A prostitute cannot, in law, be raped

For answers see over

Answers

A.15.8 a. T
         b. F—Studies in London, New York and Sydney have produced interesting data and continue at the present time.
         c. T
         d. T—Studies have shown that female prostitutes insist on a very high level of condom use among clients, but often not with their regular partners.
         e. F—A female prostitute like any other woman has the right to decline sexual intercourse even with a client. It is vital that female prostitutes who complain to physicians of being raped have standard specimens and forensic tests performed, as well as supportive counselling.

16. *Therapeutics of STDs*

Q.16.1 **The following are appropriate therapies for their associated conditions:**

a. Chlamydial infection – oxytetracycline
b. *Candida albicans* vaginosis – azithromycin
c. Bacterial vaginosis – metronidazole
d. Pharyngeal gonorrhoea – ampicillin and probenicid (as a single dose)
e. Primary syphilis – doxycycline (in a penicillin-allergic individual)

Q.16.2 **Well-recognised side effects of the tetracycline group include**

a. photosensitivity eruption
b. fixed drug eruption
c. the worsening of uraemia in patients with renal failure
d. prolongation of the QT interval on ECG
e. staining of teeth in adults

Q.16.3 **The following regimens are considered appropriate for the treatment of primary and secondary syphilis:**

a. Oral doxycycline 300 mg daily for 15 days
b. Intramuscular procaine penicillin 600,000 units for 10 days
c. Oral erythromycin 500 mg qds for 15 days
d. Intramuscular benzyl penicillin 1 mega unit daily for 15 days
e. Oral cotrimoxazole 960 mg twice daily for 2 weeks

Q.16.4 **Drugs safe for use in pregnancy include:**

a. penicillin
b. co-trimoxazole
c. acyclovir
d. clotrimazole pessaries
e. erythromycin

For answers see over

Answers

A.16.1 a. T—Erythromycin may also be used.
        b. F—Imidazole drugs such as clotrimazole are recommended in the form of pessaries or cream, oral agents such as fluconazole or itraconazole may also be used.
        c. T
        d. F—Studies have reported from 4% to 71% failure rates with single dose ampicillin and probenecid. Ciprofloxacin as a single dose is efficacious.
        e. T

A.16.2 a. T
        b. T
        c. T—Although doxycycline and minocycline are safe in this context.
        d. F
        e. F—Tetracyclines are deposited in growing bone and teeth due to calcium binding, causing staining and occasionally dental hypoplasia. They should not be prescribed to children under 12 years or to pregnant mothers.

A.16.3 a. T
        b. T
        c. T
        d. F—The slow dividing time of *Treponema pallidum* (approximately 30 hours) necessitates prolonged serum levels of penicillin. Benzyl penicillin is rapidly renally excreted and is therefore inadequate as a single daily dose.
        e. F—Co-trimoxazole is the treatment of choice for gonorrhoea in patients with suspected coincidental syphilis infection.

A.16.4 a. T
        b. F—It has an antifolate action, and also there is a risk of displacement of bilirubin from plasma proteins in the neonate if given antenatally.
        c. F—There are inadequate data on the safety of acyclovir in pregnancy.
        d. T
        e. T

Q.16.5 **Erythromycin**

  a. is active against *Chlamydia trachomatis*
  b. may cause cholestatic jaundice
  c. may be used to treat early syphilis in penicillin-allergic patients
  d. erythromycin is contraindicated in renal failure
  e. interferes with bacterial ribosomal function

Q.16.6 **Metronidazole**

  a. may produce a disulfiram like action with alcohol
  b. may cause peripheral neuropathy with prolonged therapy
  c. is the treatment of choice for *Trichomonas vaginalis* infection
  d. levels may be affected by concomitant cimetidine administration
  e. is particularly active against *Mobiluncus* spp

Q.16.7 **The following medications may cause a decrease in the effectiveness of oral contraceptives:**

  a. Rifampicin
  b. Phenytoin
  c. Griseofulvin
  d. Barbiturates
  e. Paracetamol

Q.16.8 **The following statements concerning antifungal medications are true:**

  a. Amphotericin B is active systemically after oral administration
  b. Ketaconazole may lead to hepatitis
  c. Itraconazole appears to be less hepatotoxic than ketaconazole
  d. The absorption of ketaconazole is decreased by the administration of H_2 antagonists
  e. A single dose of fluconazole is effective against vaginal candidosis

For answers see over

Answers

A.16.5 a. T
          b. T
          c. T
          d. F
          e. T

A.16.6 a. T—If alcohol is ingested this may give rise to flushing, throbbing headache, palpitations, nausea and vomiting due to accumulation of acetaldehyde in the body. Patients should therefore be advised against drinking.
          b. T
          c. T
          d. T—Cimetidine inhibits the metabolism of metronidazole and may lead to increased plasma metronidazole concentration.
          e. T

A.16.7 a. T
          b. T
          c. T
          d. T
          e. F—The enzyme induction due to rifampicin, phenytoin, griseofulvin and the barbiturates, all lead to an accelerated metabolism of both combined and progesterone only contraceptives. This may lead to reduced contraceptive effect, and patients on these medications should be advised to use other forms of contraception.

A.16.8 a. F—Amphotericin B must be administered intravenously, as it is not absorbed by the gastrointestinal tract. However, it may be used in the treatment of oral candidosis.
          b. T—This drug should be avoided in patients with deranged liver function.
          c. T
          d. T—Both ketoconazole and itraconazole depend upon the low PH of gastric fluids for their absorption. Patients on antacids, H_2 antagonists or with achlorhydria should be prescribed fluconazole.
          e. T—A single dose tablet of 150 mg is effective.

Q.16.9 **The following antiviral agents are effective against their associated viruses:**

    a. Acyclovir–varicella zoster (VCZ)
    b. Zidovudine–human immunodeficiency virus (HIV)
    c. Ganciclovir–cytomegalovirus (CMV)
    d. Acyclovir–human papilloma virus (HPV)
    e. Idoxuridine–herpes simplex virus (HSV)

Q.16.10 **Zidovudine**

    a. inhibits the reverse transcriptase of HIV I
    b. is also known as acyclovir
    c. may cause profound leukopenia
    d. produces a serum concentration which is unaffected by probenicid
    e. should not be prescribed in conjunction with aspirin

For answers see over

Answers

A.16.9   a. T—High dose oral acyclovir at a dose of 800 mg five times a day may diminish symptoms and increase healing time in shingles.
      b. T
      c. T
      d. F
      e. T

A.16.10   a. T—It inhibits the RNA-dependent DNA polymerase of HIV.
      b. F—It is also known as AZT.
      c. T—It may cause anaemia and leukopenia, and less commonly thrombocytopenia. It may also lead to a myositis with muscle weakness and raised creatine kinase levels in prolonged therapy (greater than 1 year).
      d. F—Probenecid interferes with renal excretion and may lead to increased plasma levels.
      e. F—Both paracetamol and aspirin may be prescribed in conjunction with AZT, but the manufacturers advise against prolonged co-administration.

17. *Lymphogranuloma Venereum, Chancroid and Donovanosis*

Q.17.1 *Lymphogranuloma venereum (LGV) is*

    a. caused by certain serotypes of *Chlamydia trachomatis*
    b. also known as granuloma inguinale
    c. endemic in many Pacific islands
    d. more commonly symptomatic in men than in women
    e. frequently transmitted perinatally

Q.17.2 **The initial clinical manifestation of LGV**

    a. is usually a painless indurated ulcer 0.5–1.0 cm across
    b. often goes unnoticed by the patient
    c. is usually dysuria
    d. usually develops within 3 to 12 days after exposure
    e. is usually pathognomonic and allows the diagnosis to be made on clinical grounds alone

Q.17.3 **The secondary stage of LGV**

    a. is usually associated with a non-pruritic maculopapular rash
    b. characteristically develops within 6 months of the initial lesion
    c. is usually associated with generalised lymphadenopathy
    d. typically produces tender inguinal lymphadenopathy
    e. spontaneously resolves in the majority of cases

Q.17.4 **The anorectal syndrome associated with LGV**

    a. only occurs in passive homosexual men
    b. is a form of proctocolitis and lymphatic hyperplasia
    c. may cause a tender lower abdominal mass
    d. is histologically indistinguishable from Crohn's disease
    e. frequently undergoes malignant transformation to anal cancer

For answers see over

Answers

A.17.1 a. T—LGV is usually caused by the L1, L2 or L3 serovars.
            b. F—Granuloma inguinale is a synonym for Donovanosis.
            c. F—LGV only occurs sporadically in Oceania. It is endemic in
                Africa, Asia and South America.
            d. T
            e. F

A.17.2 a. F—The primary lesion is usually a herpetiform ulcer. A
                painless indurated ulcer is more suggestive of primary
                syphilis.
            b. T
            c. F
            d. T
            e. F

A.17.3 a. F—Inguinal lymphadenopathy is the characteristic secondary
                stage.
            b. T—Although usually within the first month.
            c. F—The lymphadenopathy is usually regional.
            d. T
            e. T

A.17.4 a. F—It can occur by lymphatic spread.
            b. T
            c. T
            d. T
            e. F—Although there does appear to be a small risk of the
                development of anal cancer.

Q.17.5 In the investigation of a suspected case of LGV

a. the finding in a crush preparation of material from a bubo of intracytoplasmic organisms with bipolar chromatin staining is diagnostic
b. a Frei test is usually performed
c. the method of choice is by finding a four-fold rise in the antibody titre obtained by complement fixation
d. microimmunoflourescence tests on bubo material are unhelpful
e. chlamydia can rarely be cultured from buboes

Q.17.6 In the management of LGV

a. surgical drainage of buboes is mandatory
b. the proctocolitis usually responds well to antibiotic therapy
c. antibiotics usually have no significant effect on the diameter of any associated rectal stricture
d. penicillin is very effective
e. certain tetracyclines are effective if given for a minimum of 2 weeks

Q.17.7 Chancroid

a. is recognised more frequently in men than women
b. is more common in uncircumcised men
c. is highly prevalent in Western homosexual males
d. occurs sporadically in Western countries
e. is a rare cause of genital ulceration in African countries

Q.17.8 *Haemophilus ducreyi*

a. is the causative organism of chancroid
b. can only be successfully grown in cell cultures
c. requires nutritionally enriched media for growth
d. is serologically distinct from other *Haemophilus* species
e. probably gains entry through small skin abrasions

For answers see over

Answers

A.17.5 a. F—This is used in the diagnosis of Donovanosis.
        b. F—The Frei test is not specific to LGV and positive responses may occur after successful treatment. It is therefore no longer used.
        c. T
        d. F—Microimmunofluorescence tests are helpful, but are not generally available.
        e. F—Chlamydia can be cultured from the majority of buboes, although a wide variation in isolation has been reported.

A.17.6 a. F—Although occasionally useful.
        b. T
        c. F—Antibiotics reduce the amount of inflammatory oedema.
        d. F
        e. T—Erythromycin, chloramphenicol, rifampicin and 4-quinolones are also of value.

A.17.7 a. T
        b. T
        c. F
        d. T—Prostitutes and naval personnel are most commonly infected.
        e. F—It is a very common cause in Africa.

A.17.8 a. T
        b. F
        c. T
        d. F
        e. T

Q.17.9   Clinically apparent chancroid

a. typically has an incubation period of 4–7 days
b. is characterised by generalised lymphadenopathy
c. is usually associated with painful ulceration at sites of sexual contact
d. is not a cause of cervical ulceration
e. may be associated with spontaneously draining buboes

Q.17.10   In the diagnosis of chancroid

a. culture of material from buboes is usually helpful
b. the Frei test is helpful
c. a negative culture excludes the diagnosis
d. a fourfold rise in specific antibody titres is the usual means of diagnosis
e. false positive syphilis serology may occur

Q.17.11   The management of chancroid

a. is primarily surgical
b. frequently requires aspiration of associated buboes
c. must take the emergence of drug-resistant strains into consideration
d. must involve at least one month of antimicrobial therapy
e. may involve erythromycin or co-trimoxazole as drugs of first choice

Q.17.12   Donovanosis

a. is caused by *Calymmatobacterium granulomatis*
b. is common in India and the Caribbean
c. is associated with genital nodules which break down to form ulcers
d. responds rapidly to penicillin
e. usually responds to single-dose therapy

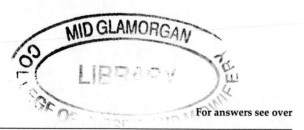

For answers see over

Answers

A.17.9 a. T
          b. F—Although painful regional lymphadenopathy is common.
          c. T
          d. F—Cervical ulceration does occur occasionally.
          e. T

A.17.10 a. T—Specific culture of *H. ducreyi* from buboes or genital ulcers is the diagnostic method of choice.
          b. F—This test was used in the diagnosis of LGV, but was abandoned in view of its lack of sensitivity and specificity.
          c. F
          d. F—Reliable serological tests are currently not available in most centres.
          e. F—There is no cross reactivity with *T. pallidum*.

A.17.11 a. F
          b. T
          c. T
          d. F—One week courses have been shown to be adequate in many cases.
          e. T

A.17.12 a. T
          b. T
          c. T
          d. F—Chloramphenicol, gentamicin and tetracyclines are some of the most effective drugs. Penicillins are not particularly helpful.
          e. F—Prolonged therapy of 3–12 weeks may be necessary.

18. *Miscellaneous: Proctitis and Molluscum Contagiosum*

Q.18.1 Anal carcinoma

    a. is exclusively a disease of those admitting to receptive anal intercourse

    b. in women is associated with an increased incidence of cervical carcinoma

    c. usually contains evidence of HPV type 16 or 18

    d. tends to arise in pre-existing anal warts

    e. typically presents with fresh rectal bleeding

Q.18.2 Proctitis

    a. caused by *Neisseria gonorrhoeae* is proof of recent receptive genitoanal intercourse

    b. due to herpes simplex virus frequently occurs in the absence of visible perianal lesions

    c. due to *Chlamydia trachomatis* is typically asymptomatic

    d. in homosexual men is usually of unknown origin

    e. should be investigated by stool examination

Q.18.3 Amoebiasis in homosexual men

    a. is usually due to *Entamoeba histolytica*

    b. is characteristically associated with fulminant bloody diarrhoea

    c. is best diagnosed by microscopic examination of a fresh stool specimen

    d. is rarely associated with disseminated infection

    e. can be effectively treated with metronidazole

Q.18.4 The prostate

    a. is congenitally absent in 5% of the male population

    b. can usually be palpated by a finger in the rectum

    c. is a major source of testosterone

    d. contributes 99% of the volume of the ejaculate

    e. tends to increase in size during life

For answers see over

Answers

A.18.1 a. F—Although there is epidemiological evidence suggesting a higher incidence in homosexual men.
      b. F
      c. T
      d. F
      e. T

A.18.2 a. F—Women may develop proctitis from passive transfer of infected secretions from the vulval area. Digitoanal and oroanal intercourse are other possible modes of acquisition.
      b. T
      c. T
      d. F—Thorough investigations will reveal a cause in up to 80% of cases, the commonest causative organism is *Neisseria gonorrhoeae*.
      e. T—Organisms such as *Campylobacter jejuni*, *Giardia lamblia* and *Shigella* spp. may be associated with proctitis.

A.18.3 a. T
      b. F—The majority of cases are asymptomatic.
      c. T
      d. T—Most infections are with non-pathogenic zymodemes.
      e. T

A.18.4 a. F
      b. T
      c. F—Testosterone is chiefly produced by the testes. Dihydrotestosterone is produced by the prostate from circulating testosterone.
      d. F
      e. T

Q.18.5   Acute bacterial prostatitis in a young man

a. is characteristically associated with systemic upset
b. is most commonly due to *Chlamydia trachomatis*
c. is usually due to ascending urethral infection
d. is best treated with penicillin, unless microbial sensitivities indicate otherwise
e. frequently requires antibiotic treatment for several weeks

Q.18.6   Chronic bacterial prostatitis

a. may be associated with urinary frequency and urgency
b. is a cause of haematospermia
c. is a cause of post-micturition dribbling
d. may result in pain in the testes
e. may lead to reduced fertility

Q.18.7   The Stamey test

a. is best performed with a full bladder
b. VB1 is the first 10 ml voided urine
c. VB2 is 10 ml from the mid-stream urine
d. VB3 follows prostatic massage
e. is strongly suggestive of bacterial colonisation of the prostate if colony former units (CFU) in VB3 are at least 10 times that of VB1 or VB2

Q.18.8   Molluscum contagiosum

a. is caused by a DNA pox virus
b. lesions may be confused with basal cell carcinoma
c. rarely causes extragenital lesions in children
d. of the genital area should lead to a search for concomitant sexually transmitted diseases
e. causes pearly white umbilicated, painful papules

For answers see over

Answers

A.18.5 a. T

         b. F—Coliforms, such as *Escherichia coli* are the commonest implicated.

         c. T

         d. F—Lipid-soluble antibiotics such as doxycycline or one of the quinolones are best.

         e. T

A.18.6 a. T

         b. T

         c. T

         d. T—The pain of chronic bacterial prostatitis is typically perineal and radiates to the genitals and groin area.

         e. T—Although evidence suggests that chronic bacterial prostatitis is an uncommon cause of male subfertility.

A.18.7 a. T

         b. T

         c. T

         d. T

         e. T

A.18.8 a. T

         b. T—Due to their pearly white appearance.

         c. F—Close physical contact is thought to facilitate their spread.

         d. T

         e. F—They are characteristically painless.

Q.18.9 **The following therapies are effective for the treatment of molluscum contagiosum:**

    a. Cryotherapy
    b. Intralesional 80% phenol
    c. Topical acyclovir
    d. Oral metronidazole
    e. Itraconazole

Q.18.10 **Molluscum contagiosum**

    a. has a unimodal age distribution
    b. may result in facial lesions in HIV-infected individuals
    c. usually has an incubation period greater than four months
    d. is commonly secondarily infected following treatment
    e. rarely undergoes spontaneous resolution

For answers see over

Answers

A.18.9 a. T
        b. T
        c. F
        d. F
        e. F

A.18.10 a. F
        b. T
        c. F
        d. T
        e. F

Informative Event T

19. Practice Exam 1

Q.19.1 **AIDS-defining illnesses in an HIV-seropositive individual include**

a. oral hairy leukoplakia
b. Kaposi's sarcoma
c. unidermatomal herpes zoster infection
d. cryptosporidial diarrhoea of two weeks' duration
e. cerebral B cell lymphoma

Q.19.2 **In the investigation of cerebral toxoplasmosis**

a. the absence of specific IgG in the serum makes the diagnosis unlikely
b. CSF IgM titres are always elevated in cerebral toxoplasmosis
c. brain biopsy should always be performed to exclude cerebral lymphoma
d. the finding of multiple ring-enhancing lesions on a CT brain scan is more suggestive of progressive multifocal leucoencephalopathy
e. India ink staining of CSF samples frequently establishes the diagnosis

Q.19.3 **Antibodies to HIV**

a. are strongly virus neutralising in asymptomatic carriers
b. can be detected in the serum of > 95% of patients with the acquired immune deficiency syndrome (AIDS)
c. are always present in people found to be carrying viable HIV
d. are only of IgG type
e. in serial titres predict the likelihood of developing full-blown AIDS

Q.19.4 **Vulval warts**

a. Have an incubation period of up to 90 days
b. Are associated with marked vaginal discharge
c. Cause inguinal lymphadenopathy
d. Are infectious to a sexual partner
e. Are not associated with abnormal cervical smears

For answers see over

Answers

A.19.1 a. F—This is classified as ARC defining.
        b. T
        c. F—Multidermatomal herpes zoster infection is an ARC defining condition.
        d. F—Cryptosporidial diarrhoea of at least four weeks duration is an AIDS defining illness.
        e. T

A.19.2 a. T—Toxoplasmosis is usually due to reactivation of old infection.
        b. F—CSF analysis is generally unhelpful.
        c. F—A diagnosis can generally be made on the basis of CT scan appearance, and response to specific antitoxoplasma therapy.
        d. F—This appearance is more characteristic of cerebral toxoplasmosis.
        e. F—This technique is used to visualise cryptococci.

A.19.3 a. F—The antibodies that have been detected to HIV are either only very weakly virus neutralising or non-virus neutralising.
        b. T
        c. F—Both false positives and false negatives occur in all the antibody tests. Infected individuals may be negative in the early infection before antibody develops, or in the late stages of AIDS when antibody levels may fall due to severe immune suppression.
        d. F—IgM antibodies are also produced, especially in the early stages of infection.
        e. F—There is no correlation.

A.19.4 a. T
        b. F—Vulval warts do not cause a marked vaginal discharge.
        c. F
        d. T
        e. F—50% per cent of patients with vulval warts have abnormal exfoliative cervical cytology.

Q.19.5 A 24-year-old girl attends your clinic. She has culture-confirmed attacks of genital herpes that recur every 3–4 weeks. She tells you she cannot bring herself to tell her new boyfriend that she has herpes but that intercourse is imminent.

She might be managed as follows:
a. She should be told to tell the boyfriend she has herpes
b. She should be told to break up with the boyfriend
c. She should be offered a 6 month course of oral acyclovir to prevent recurrences
d. She should be offered a 3 week course of oral acyclovir to prevent recurrences
e. Discuss with her why she finds it impossible to tell her boyfriend.

Q.19.6 Hepatitis B infection
a. may be associated with arthropathy in the acute phase
b. is associated with Fitz–Hugh–Curtis syndrome
c. may lead to microscopic haematuria and proteinuria
d. may be anicteric in up to 50% of acute cases
e. predisposes to hepatocellular carcinoma in chronic carriers

Q.19.7 The following are usually found in general paralysis of the insane (GPI):
a. Positive fluorescent treponemal antibody test (FTA) antibodies in the CSF
b. Cerebrovascular endarteritis
c. Cerebral atrophy
d. Hyperreflexia with upgoing plantars
e. Argyll–Robertson pupils

Q.19.8 In orogenital gonorrhoea of women
a. a high vaginal swab is the investigation of choice
b. rectal gonorrhoea co-exists in approximately 5% of patients
c. Bartholin's abscess may be a complication of infection
d. PID is unlikely to develop at the time of menstruation
e. ciprofloxacin is the treatment of choice in pregnancy

For answers see over

Answers

A.19.5 a. F—This would be a value judgement imposed on the patient
b. F—See answer a.
c. T—The frequency of attacks and the associated psychological distress would probably justify offering prophylactic therapy in this case.
d. T—Very occasionally short periods of suppressive therapy may be justified.
e. T—Once this subject is broached her anxieties and fears may be revealed.

A.19.6 a. T
b. F
c. T
d. T
e. T—Hepatitis C and D also predispose to this.

A.19.7 a. T—This is a very sensitive test of neurosyphilis in the CSF although it yields false positives in some normal patients.
b. T—This is the basic pathological defect in GPI which leads to:
c. T—Secondary cerebral atrophy.
d. T—This is the clinical result of cerebral atrophy.
e. F—These are rarely found in GPI.

A.19.8 a. F—The gonococcus preferentially colonises columnar epithelium of the cervix.
b. F—It occurs in 35%–50% of cases. Most cases are probably due to passive contamination by vaginal secretions.
c. T
d. F—Retrograde menstrual blood flow may carry *N. gonorrhoeae* to the Fallopian tubes.
e. F—Penicillin or spectinomycin is the treatment of choice.

Q.19.9 *N. gonorrhoeae* **requires for growth:**

    a. 5%–7% carbon dioxide
    b. an anaerobic atmosphere
    c. a low humidity
    d. a source of iron
    e. a temperature of 36°C

Q.19.10 *C. trachomatis*

    a. can be detected in up to 80% of cases of non-gonococcal urethritis (NGU) in heterosexual men
    b. urethritis is clinically indistinguishable from other causes of NGU
    c. infections of the male urethra are more often asymptomatic than urethral gonococcal infections
    d. is a common cause of postgonococcal urethritis in heterosexual men
    e. is frequently isolated from men with 'non-bacterial' prostatitis

Q.19.11 **Bacterial vaginosis**

    a. is always sexually transmitted
    b. is strongly associated with the development of pelvic inflammatory disease
    c. is sometimes mistaken clinically for *T. vaginalis* infection (because of the odour)
    d. occurs in females of all ages
    e. is always associated with the presence of *T. vaginalis*

Q.19.12 **In a patient with lower abdominal pain, clinical features that support a diagnosis of pelvic inflammatory disease are**

    a. pyrexia
    b. unilateral lower abdominal pain
    c. haemoglobin < 10 g/litre
    d. serum ß-human chorionic gonadotrophin (ßHCG) greater than 400 units
    e. purulent cervical discharge

For answers see over

Answers

A.19.9 a. T
         b. F
         c. F
         d. T
         e. T
N. gonorrhoeae require 5%–7% carbon dioxide, high humidity, a temperature of 36°–37°C and a source of iron for growth.

A.19.10 a. F—40% of cases of NGU are associated with *C. trachomatis.*
         b. T
         c. T
         d. T
         e. F—Evidence for the role of *C. trachomatis* is currently inconclusive.

A.19.11 a. F
         b. F
         c. T
         d. T
         e. F

A.19.12 a. T—Fever may occur but it is less pronounced in ectopic pregnancy or painful ovarian cysts.
         b. F—More common with an ectopic pregnancy.
         c. F—See answer b.
         d. F—See answer b.
         e. T—Pelvic inflammatory disease may also occur without any cervical discharge.

Q.19.13 **Drugs that may be safely given in the first trimester of pregnancy include:**
   a. ampicillin
   b. metronidazole
   c. acyclovir
   d. tetracycline
   e. erythromycin

Q.19.14 **Urethral syndrome**
   a. is defined as dysuria and frequency in the absence of bladder bacteriuria ($< 10^5$ organisms/ml urine)
   b. is defined as dysuria and frequency in the presence of bladder bacteruria ($> 10^5$ organisms/ml urine)
   c. is always associated with underlying renal pathology
   d. may be associated with the symptoms of haematuria and loin pain
   e. is also called abacterial cystitis

Q.19.15 **The conjunctivitis of adult chlamydial ophthalmia (non-trachomatous)**
   a. is usually bilateral
   b. cannot be distinguished clinically from adenovirus infection
   c. is totally unresponsive to chloramphenicol eye drops
   d. if untreated for greater than 6 months, may lead to blindness
   e. is associated with concurrent chlamydial cervical infection in 90% of women but concurrent urethral infection in only 50% of men

Q.19.16 **Lichen planus**
   a. can cause shiny, polygonal, violaceous papules on the genitals
   b. is characterised by the presence of Wickham's striae
   c. is best treated by systemic steroids
   d. is often associated with an anterior uveitis
   e. is associated with Koplik's spots in the mouth

For answers see over

Answers

A.19.13 a. T
      b. F
      c. F
      d. F
      e. T

Metronidazole has theoretical objections but these are not confirmed by clinical trials. Acyclovir has not been tested and tetracycline is not given due to its effect on the fetal teeth and bones although this effect occurs in late pregnancy.

Ampicillin and erythromycin have been used in early pregnancy with no ill effects.

A.19.14 a. T
      b. F
      c. F—The urethral syndrome is not associated with renal pathology.
      d. T
      e. T—But conventionally there may be bacteria present but not at a concentration of $> 10^5$ organisms/ml.

A.19.15 a. F—Only about one-third of cases are bilateral.
      b. T—Even with slit lamp examination it appears identical (i.e. has 'follicle' formation).
      c. F—Chloramphenicol has some antichlamydial effect but is inadequate for definitive treatment.
      d. F—Despite great similarity between trachoma (A–C) serovars and oculogenital (D–K) serovars additional factors seem to be required other than simple chlamydial infection for progression to pannus formation. Low-grade follicular conjunctivitis may, however, persist for months to years if untreated in the D–K type infection.
      e. T

A.19.16 a. T
      b. T
      c. F
      d. F
      e. F

20. *Practice Exam 2*

Q.20.1 **The following factors confer a poor prognosis in HIV infection:**

    a. Oral candidosis
    b. Seborrhoeic dermatitis
    c. A high β_2-microglobulin level
    d. A prolonged severe seroconversion illness
    e. Weight loss of greater than 10%

Q.20.2 **In the investigation of suspected PCP**

    a. blood gas analysis typically shows CO_2 retention
    b. blood cultures should be taken routinely in an attempt to culture the pneumocysts
    c. bronchoscopy is mandatory
    d. hypertonic saline may be used to induce sputum production
    e. failure to find pneumocysts on bronchoalveolar lavage specimens makes the diagnosis unlikely

Q.20.3 **Cell-mediated immunity is thought to play an important part in the eradication of the following organisms:**

    a. Mycobacteria
    b. Herpes viruses
    c. Salmonella
    d. Listeria
    e. Brucella

Q.20.4 **In the treatment of anogenital warts**

    a. podophyllin 25% should be used to treat cervical warts
    b. podophyllin should be washed off any time up to 24 h later
    c. an excess of podophyllin may be very cardiotoxic
    d. anal warts may be cut off with scissors
    e. anal warts are often the easiest to treat of all warts

For answers see over

Answers

A.20.1 a. T
           b. F
           c. T
           d. T
           e. T

A.20.2 a. F
           b. F
           c. F
           d. T
           e. T

A.20.3 a.–e. T—These are all intracellular pathogens and cell-mediated immunity therefore plays the most important role.

A.20.4 a. F—Cervical warts should not be treated with podophyllin because of the theoretical risk of oncogenicity.
           b. T—Podophyllin should be washed off any time up to 24 h after application. A test dose should be given and washed off 3 h later.
           c. F—Podophyllin is very neurotoxic in large local amounts.
           d. T—The 'scissor technique' is to infiltrate the anal area with weak adrenaline, causing the warts to be proud of the skin and then cut them off with scissors.
           e. F—Anal warts are the most difficult to treat of all warts.

Q.20.5 **The use of continuous prophylactic acyclovir**

a. is recommended for pregnant women with a history of herpes infection
b. has been shown to reduce the frequency of recurrences on cessation
c. has been shown to be safe for up to 3 years of continuous treatment in healthy individuals
d. is recommended at a dose of 400 mg qds
e. costs £4500 per year

Q.20.6 **Following acute viral hepatitis**

a. persistence of hepatitis B surface antigen for one month indicates chronic carriage
b. 5%–10% of adults become chronic carriers
c. men are more likely to become chronic carriers of hepatitis B than women
d. acute fulminant hepatitis occurs in 10% of cases of hepatitis A
e. patients should be advised to avoid alcohol for 18 months

Q.20.7 **The following are true of early syphilis:**

a. Up to 40% of patients' CSF contain *T. pallidum* prior to treatment
b. Early syphilitic hepatitis is unusual in that the alkaline phosphatase is disproportionately raised (i.e. it appears to be an obstructive hepatitis)
c. Uveitis never occurs
d. Aortic regurgitation is a known manifestation of this stage of syphilis
e. At this stage of the disease the causative organism is disseminated around the body

For answers see over

Answers

A.20.5 a. F—Acyclovir is not licensed in the UK for use in pregnancy, except with life-threatening conditions.
        b. F—No difference has been shown.
        c. T
        d. F—The recommended dose is 200 mg 4 times a day.
        e. F—The actual cost is nearer £1500.

A.20.6 a. F—Chronic carriage is defined as persisting surface antigenaemia for greater than six months.
        b. T
        c. T—Men are 2–3 times more likely to become chronic carriers.
        d. F—It occurs in less than 1% of cases.
        e. F—The need for, and duration of, abstention from alcohol is contentious.

A.20.7 a. T
        b. T
        c. F—Uveitis is rarely symptomatic but more commonly clinically silent at this stage.
        d. F—This is a manifestation of tertiary syphilis.
        e. T

Q.20.8 **The following is true about gonorrhoea:**

    a. It may be diagnosed on the basis of a Gram-stained smear of urethral exudate in about 89% of men

    b. It may be diagnosed on the basis of a Gram-stained smear of urethral exudate in about 35% of women

    c. It may be diagnosed on the basis of a Gram-stained smear of urethral and/or cervical material in up to 60% of women

    d. It may be diagnosed on the basis of a Gram-stained smear of urethral and/or cervical material in up to 35% of women

    e. Direct monoclonal antibody staining of cervical material is less sensitive than Gram-stained preparations

Q.20.9 **Selective agents used in culture media for the isolation of *Neisseria gonorrhoeae* include:**

    a. lincomycin

    b. penicillin

    c. cephalosporins

    d. trimethoprim

    e. nystatin

Q.20.10 **Pelvic inflammatory disease is:**

    a. an inflammation of the female genital tract above the level of the cervix

    b. always due to microbial infection

    c. always due to upward spread of infection from the lower genital tract

    d. always associated with cervicitis

    e. sometimes associated with perihepatitis (Fitz–Hugh–Curtis syndrome)

Q.20.11 **Infection with *T. vaginalis* is usually associated with:**

    a. a reddened vaginal mucosa

    b. the likelihood of other concurrent sexually transmitted diseases

    c. a thick white non-homogeneous discharge

    d. absence of pus cells on microscopy of vaginal fluid

    e. organisms characteristically seen on Gram-stained preparations of vaginal fluid

For answers see over

Answers

A.20.8 a. T
      b. F
      c. T
      d. F
      e. F—Monoclonal antibody stains of direct smears are more sensitive than Gram-stain preparations in females (in males of equal sensitivity).

A.20.9 a. T
      b. F
      c. F
      d. T
      e. T
Lincomycin suppresses Gram-positive organisms, trimethoprim Gram-negative organims (but only occasionally *N. gonorrhoeae*) and nystatin inhibits *Candida* spp. Penicillin would inhibit both normal flora and gonococci.

A.20.10 a. T
      b. F—Rarely other factors such as chemical or physical irritants may be responsible.
      c. F—Rarely PID can be caused by spread from an associated structure such as the appendix.
      d. F
      e. T

A.20.11 a. T—*Trichomonas vaginalis* infection usually causes inflammation.
      b. T—As *T. vaginalis* is a sexually transmitted disease, there is an association between finding it and other STDs.
      c. F—*T. vaginalis* usually results in a frothy, yellow, offensive and homogeneous discharge, unlike the thick cheesy-white discharge of candidiasis.
      d. F—The presence of an increased number of pus cells on microscopy of the vaginal fluid reflects the inflammatory response to *T. vaginalis*.
      e. F—Mobile trichomonads are seen on examination of the 'wet' film of vaginal fluid seen on either dark-field or light microscopy. They will be missed on a fixed Gram stain.

Q.20.12 Recognised long-term sequelae of PID include:

a. chronic pelvic pain
b. tubal infertility
c. recurrent early pregnancy loss
d. increased risk of ectopic pregnancy
e. anovulatory cycles

Q.20.13 The following is true of acute anaphylaxis after penicillin (ampicillin) treatment:

a. The most important therapeutic action is to give 100 mg i.v. hydrocortisone as a bolus
b. The most important therapeutic action is to give 5 ml 1:10,000 adrenaline intramuscularly into the pectoral muscles
c. It may follow oral amoxycillin
d. It may present with the patient feeling they have been killed by the doctor or nurse who gave the injection of procaine penicillin
e. It may lead to bronchospasm

Q.20.14 Genital ulcers

a. in industrialised Western countries are more common than urethritis or vaginitis
b. are usually caused by herpes simplex virus infection in Western countries
c. may be caused by syphilitic infection
d. are often the result of chancroid in Asia and Africa
e. may be caused by drug therapy

Q.20.15 *C. albicans* in the vagina

a. is found in about one-third of normal women
b. may cause dysuria
c. is characterised by an offensive fishy discharge
d. raises the vaginal pH above 5
e. should always be treated

For answers see over

Answers

A.20.12 a. T
            b. T
            c. F
            d. T
            e. T

Chronic lower abdominal pain is sometimes a result of pelvic infection and this is not always due to reinfection. Infertility after PID is due to tubal damage, which in turn leads to increased risk of ectopic pregnancy. The menstrual cycle is not affected and the cause of recurrent early pregnancy loss has yet to be established, although postendometritis intrauterine adhesions have been suggested.

A.20.13 a. F—The most important first move is to give adrenaline. This may be life-saving. Antihistamine and steroids may be given after this.
            b. T—See answer a.
            c. T—Acute anaphylaxis has been reported to occur within 30 min of oral ingestion of amoxycillin.
            d. F—This is the procaine reaction – not anaphylaxis.
            e. T

A.20.14 a. F
            b. T
            c. T
            d. T
            e. T

A.20.15 a. T
            b. T
            c. F
            d. F
            e. F

Vaginitis is usually caused by *C. albicans* or *T. vaginalis* and less commonly by streptococci. It may also result from local chemical irritation.

C. albicans colonises the vagina of a large proportion of normal women some of whom may be asymptomatic and do not require treatment. The pH is not raised.

Q.20.16 Behçet's syndrome

    a. is characterised by the presence of oral and genital ulceration
    b. is associated with arthritis in over 50% of cases
    c. only occurs in patients from Mediterranean and Eastern countries
    d. is associated with HLA B5, HLA B12 and HLA B27
    e. is best treated by radiotherapy

For answers see over

Answers

A.20.16 a. T

b. T—There is usually symmetrical involvement of the small peripheral joints.

c. F—Although it is commoner in these areas as well as in Japan.

d. T

e. F—Treatment of choice for acute episodes is steroids.

References

References

General References

Adler MW (ed) (1988) Diseases in the homosexual male. (Bloomsbury Series in Clinical Science.) Springer-Verlag, Berlin

Adler MW (ed) (1990) ABC of sexually transmitted diseases. BMA, London

Csonka GW, Oates JK (1990) Sexually transmitted diseases. A textbook of genitourinary medicine. Balliere Tindall, London

Foster SM, Harris JRW (ed) (1991) Recent advances in sexually transmitted diseases and AIDS, 4. Churchill Livingstone, Edinburgh

Hare MJ (ed) (1988) Genital tract infection in women. Churchill Livingstone, Edinburgh

Holmes KK, Mardh PA, Sparling PF, Weisner PH (1990) Sexually transmitted diseases, 2nd edn, McGraw-Hill, New York

Oriel JD, Harris JRW (1986) Recent advances in sexually transmitted diseases, 3. Churchill Livingstone, Edinburgh

Ridley CM (ed) (1988) The vulva. Churchill Livingstone, Edinburgh

Wright DJM (1988) Immunology of sexually transmitted diseases. Kluwer Academic Publishers, Dordrecht

Bacterial Vaginosis

Easmon CSF, Hay PE, Ison CA (1992) Bacterial vaginosis: a diagnostic approach. Genitourin Med 68:134–138

Larsson PG, Platz-Christensen JJ, Sundstrom E (1992) Is bacterial vaginosis a sexually transmitted disease? Int J STD AIDS 2:362–364

Thomason JL, Gelbart SM, Broekhuizen FF (1989) Advances in the understanding of bacterial vaginosis. J Reprod Med 34:581–587

Chlamydial Disease

Darougar S (ed) (1983) Chlamydial disease. Br Med Bull 39:107–203

Oriel JD, Ridgway GL (1982) Genital infection by *Chlamydia trachomatis*. Arnold, London

Radcliffe KW, Rowen D, Mercey DE, Mumtaz G, Ridgway GL, Robinson AJ, Bingham JS (1990) Is a test of cure necessary following treatment for cervical infection with *Chlamydia trachomatis*? Genitourin Med 66:444–446

Taylor-Robinson D, Thomas BJ (1991) Laboratory techniques for the diagnosis of chlamydial infections. Genitourin Med 67:256–266

Woolley PD (1990) Recent advances in non-gonococcal urethritis: pathogenesis, investigation and treatment. Int J STD AIDS 1:157–160

References

Cervical Neoplasia and Colposcopy

Campion MJ, Singer A, Clarkson PK, McCance DJ (1985) Increased risk of cervical neoplasia in the consorts of men with penile condylomata acuminata. Lancet i:943–946

Cartier (1977) Practical colposcopy. Karger, Basel

Editorial (1992) Cervical cancer screening: quest for automation. Lancet i:963–964

Oriel JD (1990) Human papillomaviruses and genital neoplasia: the changing scene. Int J STD AIDS 1:7–9

Singer A (ed) (1990) Premalignant lesions of the lower genital tract. In: Baggish MS (ed) Clinical practice of gynecology. Elsevier, New York, No. 2

Singer A (ed) (1991) Clinical practice of gynaecology: premalignant lesions of the lower genital tract. Elsevier, New York

Singer A, Walker PG, McCance DJ (1984) Genital wart virus infections: nuisance or potentially lethal? Br Med J 288:735–737

Stanley M (1990) Genital papillomaviruses, polymerase chain reaction and cervical cancer. Genitourin Med 66:415–417

Walker PG, Singer A, Dyson JL, Shah KV, Wilters J, Coleman DV (1983) Colposcopy in the diagnosis of papillomavirus infection of the uterine cervix. Br J Obstet Gynaecol 90:1082–1086

Gonorrhoea

Ison CA (1990) Methods of diagnosing gonorrhoea. Genitourin Med 66:453–459

Mindel A (1990) The changing pattern of antibiotic resistance of Neisseria gonorrhoeae. Genitourin Med 66:55–56

Morton RS (1977) Gonorrhoea (Major Problems in Dermatology Series – 9). Saunders, London

Hepatitis

Boag F (1991) Hepatitis B: heterosexual transmission and vaccination strategies. Int J STD AIDS 2:318–324

Gilson RJC (1992) Sexually transmitted hepatitis: a review. Genitourin Med 68:123–129

Piot P, Andre F (eds) (1990) Hepatitis B – a sexually transmitted disease in heterosexuals. Elsevier, Amsterdam

References

Genital Herpes

Corey L, Holmes KK (1983) Genital herpes simplex virus infections. Current concepts in diagnosis, therapy and prevention. Ann Intern Med 98:973–983

Mercey DE, Mindel A (1991) Preventing neonatal herpes? Genitourin Med 67:1–2

Mindel A (1989) Herpes simplex virus. Springer-Verlag, Berlin

Mindel A, Weller IV, Faherty A, Sutherland S, Hindley D, Fiddian AP, Adler MW (1984) Prophylactic oral acyclovir in recurrent genital herpes. Lancet ii:57–59

AIDS and Immunology

Adler MW (1991) ABC of AIDS, 2nd edn, BMA, London

Cohen PT, Sande MA, Volberding PA (eds) (1990) The AIDS knowledge base. Massachusetts Medical Publishing Group, Waltham

Farthing C, Brown SE, Staughton RC (1988) A colour atlas of AIDS and HIV disease, 2nd edn, Wolfe Medical, London

Levy JA (ed) (1991) AIDS 1990. A year in review. Current Science, Philadelphia

Parkin JM, Peters BS (1991) Differential diagnosis in AIDS – a colour guide. Wolfe Medical, Aylesbury

Strang J, Stimson G (eds) (1990) AIDS and drug misuse. Routledge, London

Youle M, Clarbour J, Wade P, Farthing C (1989) AIDS therapeutics in HIV disease. Churchill Livingstone, Edinburgh

Pelvic Inflammatory Disease

Hare J (1990) Pelvic inflammatory disease: current approaches and ideas. Int J STD AIDS 1:393–400

Jacobson L, Westrom L (1969) Objectivised diagnosis of acute PID. Am J Obstet Gynecol 105:1088–1098

Mardh PA (1980) An overview of infectious agents of salpingitis, their biology and recent advances in methods of detection. Am J Obstet Gynecol 138:933–951

Stacey CM, Barton SE, Singer A (1991) Pelvic inflammatory disease. In: Studd, J. (ed) Progress in Obstetrics and Gynaecology Volume 9. Churchill Livingstone, Edinburgh

References

Prostatitis

De la Rosette JJ, Debruyne FM (1991) Nonbacterial prostatitis: a comprehensive review. Urol Int 46(2):121–125

Krieger JN (1984) Prostatitis syndromes: pathophysiology, differential diagnosis and treatment. Sex Transm Dis 11:100–112

Thin RN (1991) The diagnosis of prostatitis: a review. Genitourin Med 67(4):279–283

Psychosexual

Bancroft J (1989) Human sexuality and its problems, 2nd edn. Churchill Livingstone, Edinburgh

Frost DP (1985) Recognition of hypochondriasis in a clinic for sexually transmitted diseases. Genitourin Med 61:133–137

Ross MW (1986) Psychovenereology: personality and lifestyle factors in sexually transmitted diseases in homosexual men. Praeger, New York

Syphilis

King A, Nicol C (1980) Venereal diseases, 4th edn, Balliere Tindall, London, pp 1–171

Kirchner JT (1991) Syphilis – an STD on the increase. Am Fam Physician 44:843–854

Tramont EC (1991) Controversies regarding the natural history and treatment of syphilis in HIV disease. AIDS Clin Rev:97–107

Zenker PN, Rolfs RT (1990) Treatment of syphilis, 1989. Rev Infect Dis 12:S590–S609

Family Planning

Guillebaud J (1989) Contraception: your questions answered. Churchill Livingstone, Edinburgh

HPV Infection

Scoular A (1991) Choosing equipment for treating genital warts in genitourinary medicine clinics. Genitourin Med 67:413–419

Thin RN (1992) Meatoscopy: a simple technique to examine the distal anterior urethra in men. Int J STD AIDS 1:21–23

Von Krogh G, Rylander E (eds) (1989) GPV1: genitoanal papilloma virus infection. Sweden Conpharm AB, Karlstad

Candida

White DJ, Emens M, Shamanesh M (1991) Recurrent vulvovaginal candidosis. Int J STD AIDS 2:235–239

Trichomonas

Hammill HA (1989) *Trichomonas vaginalis*. Obstet Gynecol Clin North Am 16:531–540

Tropical Infections

Schmid GP (1990) Treatment of chancroid. Rev Infect Dis 12:5580–5589
Vandyck E, Piot P (1992) Laboratory techniques in the investigation of chancroid, lymphogranuloma venereum and donovanosis. Genitourin Med 68:130–133

Dermatology

Rook A, Wilkinson DS, Ebling FJG, Champion RH, Burton JL (eds) (1986) Textbook of Dermatology. Blackwell, Oxford